B.A.R.D. in the Practice

A guide for family doctors to consult efficiently, effectively and happily

Ed Warren

General Practitioner, Sheffield
GP Trainer, Barnsley Vocational Training Scheme

Fore\

M
(

The Library, Ed & Trg Centre   KTW
Tunbridge Wells Hospital at Pembury
Tonbridge Rd, Pembury
Kent TN2 4QJ
01892 635884 and 635489

Phili

Forme Books must be returned/renewed by the last date shown

1LL / SBR

3 JUL 2006   DISCARDED

Rad(
Oxfo

Radcliffe Publishing Ltd
18 Marcham Road
Abingdon
Oxon OX14 1AA
United Kingdom

www.radcliffe-oxford.com
Electronic catalogue and worldwide online ordering facility.

British Library Cataloguing in Publication Data

A catalogue record for this book is available from the British Library.

ISBN 1 85775 665 7

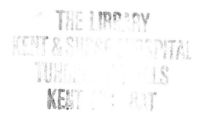
Typeset by Anne Joshua & Associates, Oxford
Printed and bound by TJ International Ltd, Padstow, Cornwall

Contents

Foreword

As a practising GP, I am constantly aware of the need to maintain rigour in clinical practice and to be accountable for my decisions in the NHS. I also know that clinical general practice is becoming more challenging. Both patients and doctors have increasing expectations of the consultation. I am all too aware from my work in clinical governance that some GPs get into difficulty as a result of dysfunctional consultations which result in complaints.

So it is my belief that we need to do more to support GPs in improving – even further – their professional consultation and communication skills. It never ceases to amaze me how in a relatively short space of time – usually ten minutes – a skilled GP can achieve some fantastic results. This is an undervalued aspect of general practice. The proven benefits of primary care are essentially derived from the consultation – the 'life and soul' of general practice.

Anything that might help GPs to deliver this goal is to be welcomed. This book will appeal to any GP who wants to get better outcomes from their consultations and who wants to feel 'less pressurised'. It comes from a practising GP who has obviously thought a lot about the issues. When I first read about BARD I became sufficiently interested to invite Ed Warren to run a workshop in the Leicester Faculty of the RCGP. This was a novel approach that was nonetheless practical, achievable and realistic.

He has developed and refined the BARD model even further by documenting the key issues and analysing the ethical dimension. BARD is a step-by-step guide for GPs to improve both their consulting skills and their well-being. Just as a cardiac surgeon will refine their surgical skills, GPs need to hone and refine their main intervention, which is the consultation. I am sure that in the future there will be a requirement for consultations to have more structure, with an emphasis on outcomes. GPs will have to learn and use strategies that enable them to get the best possible clinical results.

I am also interested in the issue of professional 'happiness' and factors that contribute to burnout. I am convinced that so-called 'difficult consultations' – often with resultant complaints – are a major source of stress among GPs. BARD emphasises the importance of maintaining good professional relationships. Both doctors and patients have agendas that need to be addressed in a consultation. I know that a notable proportion of patients still leave the doctor's office with at least one significant question unanswered. After all, preventing a breakdown in the doctor–patient relationship is a key aspect of good general practice.

As chairman of the RCGP my goal is very simple – to bring in a new standard for general practice throughout the UK. This means better quality and improved safety of patient care. This book is therefore a welcome addition to the library of consultation skills. I hope that it will stimulate debate and raise awareness of the art and science of the consultation. It will be a valuable resource for enabling GPs to achieve better doctor–patient relationships.

Mayur Lakhani FRCGP
Chairman of Council
Royal College of General Practitioners
September 2005

Foreword

The consultation is central to what we general practitioners do. It is our operating theatre and our laboratory bench. Expectations of consultations keep rising. Our expectations of ourselves and our colleagues are heightened year by year. However, the expectations of our patients are also increasing, perhaps faster than ours.

The development of consulting skills has been phenomenal. As we have evolved from the patient–child to adult–adult model of relationships, the demands on our skills have grown. It is no longer enough, if it ever was, to lay down the law. We must now engage with each patient, persuading and supporting their choices and decisions.

Perhaps the most dramatic change has been in the provision of information in such a way that patients can use it effectively. We provide it verbally and in writing. Patients seek it from friends, relatives, the media and the Internet. Increasingly we are dealing with a sophisticated and informed population who demand that they should take control of their healthcare.

Yet we still have a long way to go. Information alone is not enough. An informed consumer of healthcare needs to be educated in how to use information to make choices, and then supported in carrying through their decisions. This is no small task, and many feel that the 'health system' acts on them, not with them. Many patients feel very disempowered.

Support for good decision making needs to be timely (advice on how to handle a temperature in a child with diabetes cannot wait until the morning), accurate (messages are all too often inconsistent) and culturally appropriate. General practitioners cannot offer all of this, but they can play a pivotal role.

Patients will only take responsibility for decisions about their health if they are given permission and encouragement to do so. Effective consultations do just that. A general practitioner's approval – demonstrated by attitude as well as by words – is often all that is required.

How might we achieve this? There are many models of consulting that have been promoted over the years, and each has its merits. However, this excellent book sets out a new way of looking at consultations, namely the BARD system (which stands for behaviour, aims, room and dialogue). This easy-to-assimilate method will help us all to be more effective partners in the centrepiece of general practice, namely the consultation.

Mike Pringle
Professor of General Practice, University of Nottingham
GP Leader, NPfIT
September 2005

Foreword

The essence of general practice is the consultation. One of the intriguing aspects of medicine is that wherever in the world consultations are conducted or observed, they are surprisingly recognisable. This is despite differences in geography, location, language, culture, expectations and demands.

The context of primary care provision is changing quite quickly at present, not just in the UK but in many other countries as well. The changes in patients' understanding and expectations, economic, social and political pressures, new medical technology and treatment options are all affecting the provision and delivery of care.

There are well-founded concerns about the often erroneous assumption that the family doctor's work can be undertaken by those without medical education, training and experience, and that the work can be fragmented into discreet, easily defined parcels of care.

The research evidence increasingly demonstrates that such approaches are naive and misguided. The work of a family doctor is highly complex and skilled. The key tool for both the patient and the doctor is the consultation.

In the midst of changes in healthcare provision, the vital role of the family doctor must not be lost or diluted.

This book addresses not just the art of the consultation, but also the issue of why the consultation needs to be analysed, understood and developed. In doing so it reaffirms the important values of family medicine within a healthcare system for the benefit of individual patients and their families.

Philip R Evans
Former President of WONCA Region Europe
September 2005

Preface

The essential unit of medical practice is the occasion when, in the intimacy of the consulting room or sick room, a person who is ill or believes himself to be ill seeks the advice of a doctor whom he trusts. This is a consultation, and all else in the practice of medicine derives from it.

J Spence (1960)[1]

We have left undone those things which we ought to have done, and we have done those things which we ought not to have done, and there is no health in us . . .

Book of Common Prayer

What would induce a middle-aged family doctor of sober habits and previous good behaviour to want to write another book about the family practice consultation? Being a family doctor is undoubtedly the best job in the world. You meet great people and learn lots of exciting and interesting things. There are not many who would argue that family medicine is irrelevant, unnecessary or uncivilised. Primary care family medicine is the best way known to bring healthcare to the maximum number of people with the maximum efficiency. But if family medicine is so wonderful, why are so many family doctors anxious, depressed, addicted to drugs or suicidal?

Consulting is the core activity of family doctors, just as it was nearly half a century ago when Spence wrote the above words. The good things that result from family medicine nearly all originate in a consultation, and for a family doctor consulting should be a major source of professional satisfaction and sustenance. An attempt to work out why family doctors are such a sickly bunch must perforce ask whether there is anything in the way in which they consult that is making them ill. Perhaps more pressingly, can family doctors learn to consult in a way that is less damaging to themselves?

As a practitioner with a few miles on the clock, I think that my consulting is pretty good. My outcomes are on a par with those of my colleagues, and from the patients' point of view I get fewer complaints and more pressure for appointments in my surgeries than most. Yet when I measure my performance against the MRCGP video criteria – probably the most influential and authoritative criteria available in the UK – I consistently fail, with sins of both omission and commission, as the *Book of Common Prayer* would have it. My consultations do not contain all of the things that they should contain, and they contain lots of things that do not appear in the MRCGP or indeed any other criteria. Is there something wrong with me, or with the consulting models that I am aspiring to follow?

I want to express myself and my personality through my work. My work is important to me, and I would be unhappy if I thought that what I did all day was inconsistent with my principles and character. I want to be me, not a part-time family doctor and a part-time person. I think that the relationships I build up at work between myself as a person and the patients I work with as people are an important part of the therapy, and that there is scope within family medicine for an infinite variety of practitioners to build unique relationships with an infinite variety of patients. However, I have spent very little time examining my principles and values, and considering what sort of family doctor I want to be. So much of a family doctor's life is demand-led that it is almost impossible to determine which motivations are your own and which are imposed. Many family doctors go through life just 'doing their duty' – a strategy which brings its own satisfaction but provides little insight into personal motivations. Family doctors ought to have a clear view of what they want to be, so that they can behave accordingly and plan the necessary direction of their professional progress.

Consultation techniques, skills and attitudes have changed and continue to change, reflecting both the accumulating evidence and changes in political and social realities. Deriving new skills for new situations should demand our most pressing attention. But must we re-invent the wheel? Other people 'out there' are confronting similar problems and may have answers that a family doctor could pinch. The obvious professional group with particular expertise in communication and translating motivation into behaviour is actors. Might the theory of acting provide some good ideas for consulting in family practice? While I was writing this book, the British Government decided that general practitioners no longer exist, and that henceforth they should be known as *primary care performers*. What more compelling evidence could there be that the day of the actor/family doctor has arrived?

My task, then, is to devise a model of the family medicine consultation that is practical and usable, that takes into account a family doctor's personality and principles, that (where appropriate) learns lessons from other professional groups who work in the same general area, and that goes some way towards reducing the stress that family doctors encounter. Whether BARD fulfils this brief, I leave you to decide. I hope that the use of BARD will help family doctors to consult efficiently, effectively and happily, and promote a 'win–win' collaborative relationship with their patients. If nothing else, I hope this book will highlight some of the consulting problems that family doctors currently have, and promote discussion about how they might be resolved.

Ed Warren
September 2005

Reference

1. Spence J (1960) The need for understanding the individual as part of the training and function of doctors and nurses. In: *The Purpose and Practice of Medicine*. Oxford University Press, London.

Acknowledgements

This book has been several years in gestation, and I have asked for many favours from people who have better things to do. So I have accumulated a few debts of gratitude that need to be repaid. To Michelle Gutteridge – Leicester's simulated patient par excellence, who kept me on track when I thought that the idea of acting in a consultation solved all my problems – many thanks. To Mayur Lakhani – who wrote a foreword and got me to take an RCGP workshop in Leicester, thereby prompting invaluable feedback – many thanks. To Andy Baxter – former editor of *Update*, who published a series of articles on BARD in his esteemed organ – many thanks. To Andrea Wallace – my family practice trainee, who did a dry run of many of the training exercises – many thanks. To Amar Rughani – with whom I share a practice, for constant encouragement, rude comments about my detractors, and selfless proofreading – many thanks. To Mike Pringle and Philip Evans – for writing the other forewords – many thanks. And to my wife Dee, and daughters Kate and Jenny – who have grown up while I have been messing about with BARD – it's all over, so I can be reintroduced into the washing-up rota.

Ed Warren

Note on the text

To save having to write 'he and she', 'his and hers' and so on, repeatedly, for convenience family doctors will be referred to throughout as female. This does not exclude males, and simply reflects what will imminently be commonest in UK primary care. For contrast, and again not for reasons of exclusion, patients will be referred to as male.

I have referred to 'family doctors' throughout, but it will be clear that most of the material is based on the experience of a UK general practitioner (GP).

Chapter 1

An introduction to BARD

We've come a long way

Family doctors should really feel very proud of themselves. The rate of improvement in the standard of primary care consulting is nothing short of remarkable. A patient of the 1950s would scarcely recognise what goes on today. The science has changed – there are now many more treatments available from primary care for more conditions, and also more reasons to refer patients to hospital for increasingly sophisticated investigations and procedures. There is more emphasis on prevention and chronic disease monitoring than ever before. Patients spend more time in each visit to their family doctor in order to accommodate the extra things that now go on in a normal primary care consultation.

Another change that the patient of the 1950s would notice is the increasing trend for family doctors to work in teams, and the organisational changes that this has required. In the past, where a family doctor worked at all with non-medical people, it was on the assumption that the family doctor was in charge and told the others what to do. Now, in contrast, family practice could not survive without teamworking, and nearly all family doctors accept that in many instances a non-medical team member is the best person to provide the service. In the UK, most out-of-hours care is delivered by workers who have nothing to do with the patient's family doctor practice. Most preventive work and an increasing amount of urgent work is dealt with by nursing colleagues, and more consulting is going on over the telephone and the Internet.

Yet despite these considerable structural alterations, the major change that the patient of the 1950s would notice is in the attitude and behaviour of their family doctor.

- Fifty years ago, medical paternalism was considered to be a legitimate consultation strategy. Patients had a duty to do as they were told by their family doctor, and nearly everyone was familiar with phrases like 'doctor's orders' and 'doctor knows best'. 'Poor compliance' was the phrase used for patients who would not do as they were told and did not take their medicines properly. The case is now firmly established for patient empowerment – many (but not all) patients are most content when they are active and informed participants in the planning and progress of their care.[1]
- In 1976, Byrne and Long found that many consultations never got to first base – the family doctor never found out why the patient had come – and showed how inflexible most family doctors were in using their consultation skills.[2] A mere three decades later, all family doctors in training in the UK have their communication techniques subjected (on video) to the closest external

scrutiny. The major UK postgraduate family doctor qualifications all require candidates to be assessed on their consulting skills.

- The currently established ideas about what constitutes a good consultation have almost all been developed in the last 30 years or so. Considering the antiquity of the medical profession, this represents a staggering effort by family doctors to learn new skills (and discard old ones) in order to improve the quality of their performance.

Changes of such speed and magnitude might be expected to have a distressing effect on primary care patients, especially on those who use the services a lot and who have memories of how things used to be. However, this has not happened. Taking the UK as an example, a MORI survey in 2004 reported that 92% of the public trusted doctors to tell the truth and were satisfied with the way that doctors do their job. These figures were higher than for any other professional group, and higher than they were in the previous survey in 1983.[3] Further evidence comes from the data on complaints. In the UK the number of complaints about doctors has certainly risen in recent years,[4] but still only a tiny minority of family doctor consultations result in a patient complaint. It is a tribute to the skills of workers in primary care that they have been able to achieve considerable change and at the same time kept the goodwill of their patients.

The challenges

Ideas about primary care consulting continue to develop. As new ideas emerge, so family doctors must adjust their consulting performance. They have shown themselves to be ready and willing to respond to such challenges. It would be wrong to think that the observed changes and improvements in family doctor consulting skills are just a reaction to changing political, social and organisational circumstances. The most important engine driving forward developments in family doctor consulting is the fact that individual family doctors want to improve, to 'do it better' next time.

Changing social attitudes towards professionalism and professional groups necessitate new consultation skills. The medical profession is no longer regarded as what Goffman termed in 1959 a 'sacred team' immune from criticism.[5] It is no longer acceptable for medicine to be closed and internally regulated, without outside scrutiny. Changing social realities inevitably lead to changes in the way that family doctors are accredited as being fit to practise. This is not a challenge just for medical professionals – many other professional groups are obliged to cope with very similar problems. However, if family doctors are no longer members of a 'sacred team', immune from criticism, then the power relationships (the relative authority in the relationship as perceived by the participants) within individual consultations alter, and family doctors must adjust their performance accordingly.

Changing attitudes towards the rights of consumers of services also present consulting challenges. Patients and society at large are ever more vociferous about what they want and expect from a family doctor consultation. The promotion of clinical guidelines (and in some instances their production) by authoritative bodies such as governments provides a framework of standards that patients can expect by right. If her patient's cholesterol or blood pressure is not in the target range, a family doctor can expect that patient to be banging on the door and asking why. People generally expect to be satisfied when they are consumers of a service, and will not be automatically content with what they are given. They are less prepared than in the past to tolerate rudeness or a sub-optimal clinical performance, and are more likely to complain when offended.[4] Of course family doctors (with a tiny number of dishonourable exceptions) do not go out of their way to behave badly or provide poor clinical care, and never have done so, but they must now reflect more carefully on the consequences if their performance is perceived to be not up to the required standard.

Developments in technology present consulting challenges. If more consultations are to take place by telephone or over the Internet, then skills appropriate to such developments need to be learned by family doctors. The authority of the medical profession has traditionally depended (in part) on doctors knowing more about medicine than their patients. However, medical information is no longer exclusive information, and is potentially accessible to anyone with a modem. The extent of medical information also makes it abundantly clear that no doctor can possibly know everything there is to know. An extra problem for family doctors is that the specialised knowledge of family medicine, and the special qualities of the generalist, although vital to the success of healthcare delivery, are still often considered the poor relations of all the sexy things that go on in hospitals.

Organisational changes within primary care require new consulting skills from family doctors, and the pace of organisational change shows no sign of slowing. Where nurses provide more first-up patient care, the family doctor has to assume a role as a second-line practitioner and second opinion. Her consultations will be concerned with more complex medical problems, the ones that the nurse has not been able to deal with. Sometimes she may need considerable powers of diplomacy to sort out situations where there has been a problem with the nurse–patient interaction. It is not at all clear that traditional consulting methods will be appropriate to deal with such changes. The work of the family doctor of the future will certainly be more intensive, and it is debatable whether she will be able to sustain the quality of her performance for the number of hours of the traditional family doctor's working day.

Organisational changes that superficially appear to be patient-friendly are also not neutral in the consulting challenges they can present. Primary care should be readily available to those who need it, but it is often only possible to make an assessment of whether a patient's 'want' was just a want or a need after a consultation. Patients consult a doctor when they are concerned about something, and it is the doctor's job to translate that concern into a diagnosis and management plan. Thus better attention to patient need is usually interpreted as shorter waits to see a doctor. Such a process means either having more available family doctors (which for many practical reasons is not going to happen, and certainly not quickly), or offering patients a consultation with a non-doctor – a process that presents its own challenges (see above). If patients present with their illnesses at an earlier stage, then primary care workers need to get better at recognising and managing those illnesses at an unfamiliar earlier stage. If a primary care consultation is more readily available, it may be regarded as less important by patients, further altering the power relationships within the ensuing consultation. The consultation techniques that family doctors use depend in part on the authority they have in relation to their patients. If this balance is disrupted, it is not certain that those same techniques will continue to work.

Healthy solutions

It is tempting to seek solutions to new challenges by doing more of the same – by the expansion of tried and tested methods. This is the Boxer approach to problems (the horse from Orwell's *Animal Farm*) – 'I will work harder'. It didn't work for Boxer and it is unlikely to work for family doctors. When a significant challenge presents itself, it is often necessary to go back to basics to find a solution, and not be limited by how things have always been done. Such a 'root-and-branch' review is not always needed, but such an option must always be on any agenda for change.

Any solutions adopted by family doctors for their problems must not jeopardise their own health and well-being. A family doctor who has retired early, is off sick or is dead is unlikely to deliver good care. The track record is not very good – the mental health of family doctors in the UK is reported to be poor, significantly worse than the average for the general population,[6,7] and (intriguingly) also significantly worse than the average for the patients for whom they are caring. Family doctors spend a lot of their time consulting, probably more time than on any other single professional activity. The consultation is also central to the care delivery process, the job for which all family doctors have been trained. Each consultation should be a source of intellectual and professional satisfaction and self-esteem for a family doctor. It need not and must not be just another reason to feel guilty and frustrated.

Consultation models

A number of authoritative, elegant, well-researched and thought-provoking consulting models are available – a 'toolbox' of valuable insights into the day-to-day experience of work as a family doctor. Some of the more comprehensive consultation models are published as assessment devices. Because they are comprehensive, these models are more likely to be aspired to by family doctors (even if they are not being formally assessed), and provide a benchmark against which family doctors will inevitably measure themselves. The fact that they are designed for assessment purposes does not mean that these are any less important as consultation models.

The most widely used consultation model for training and assessment in UK family practice is the one implied by the video module of the examination for Membership of the Royal College of General Practitioners (MRCGP), a model which is also used for Membership by Assessment of Performance (MAP) and Fellowship by Assessment (FBA) (*see* Appendix 1.1 for details of this model). The model is derived from the suggestions for teaching consultation skills through the use of video contained in *The Consultation: an approach to teaching and learning* by Pendleton *et al.*[8] Like many of the other models in widespread use, it is primarily 'task based' in so far as it sets out a list of things that family doctors ought to be able to do when consulting.

All consultation models must be considered as 'work in progress'. *Skills for Communicating with Patients* by Silverman, Kurtz and Draper[9] has gone to a second edition, updated in the light of emerging evidence and understanding. *The Doctor's Communication Handbook* by Tate is now in its fourth edition.[10] *The Inner Consultation* by Neighbour[11] went into a second edition in 2004, the first edition having been published in 1987, and it remains to be seen whether this later edition will be current for as long. Authoritative as the MRCGP model is, it is nevertheless subject to an ongoing process of update and refinement, so the assessment criteria change year by year. The context in which consulting occurs is constantly altering, and a model must alter as well if it is to remain valid. New insights into consulting are emerging – it would be complacent to assume that the last word on the family doctor consultation has already been written.

The number of tasks required by a task-based consultation model inevitably limits its usefulness in day-to-day consulting. *The Consultation* suggests that there are seven tasks which need to be completed in each consultation, but when one comes to look at the 'consultation map' the number has mysteriously jumped to 11 tasks, and the suggested consultation rating scale contains 14 items.[8] There are four areas of consulting competence for Summative Assessment, the standard final assessment in UK family doctor training. The MRCGP video performance criteria 2005 weigh in with 14 items, although admittedly this is down from 21 in 2003.[12] The Calgary–Cambridge model identifies 71 separate consultation skills.[9] And the original edition of *The Inner Consultation*[11] suggests five main tasks, 58 sub-tasks and 169 sub-sub-tasks that are potentially worthy of attention during each consultation (I know because I have counted them). Not for nothing has the family doctor consultation been described as having 'exceptional potential.'[13]

Clearly it is not remotely possible to complete 169 tasks in every consultation. Any family doctor who tried to do so would end up a nervous wreck – the more tasks there are to be performed, the less chance there is of completing them all and the greater the potential sense of inadequacy and failure. Trying to complete all of the tasks suggested by these models may well be damaging to a family doctor's mental health. Even taking the view that every family doctor consultation is in fact one of a series, and in the UK every patient spends an average of 47 minutes each year with a family doctor,[14] the number of tasks which can be achieved is still limited. Patients also have an annoying habit of developing new problems between consultations, so that some tasks have to be repeated.

John was a bright young thing who had done well at school and passed all of his exams. Going into medicine seemed the best way of using his undoubted talents, and a career in family practice was clearly the optimum way of bringing the most benefit to the largest number of people. He recognised at an early stage just how vital it was to consult proficiently and communicate with patients, and so was desperate to do well in his MRCGP video module.

As he was completing his family doctor training, John studied the MRCGP video performance criteria, and convinced himself that they were all necessary and relevant to every consultation. However, when he tried to make his video he found it almost impossible to shoehorn every criterion into every consultation, and if he did manage it then the consultation

Continued

invariably ran beyond its allotted time. Also, when he came to review the tapes, he looked like a ferret on amphetamines – gone was the calm assurance he had worked so hard to portray. He was getting quite depressed about this until he realised that all of his fellow learners were having exactly the same problems, and a couple had given up doing the exam as a consequence.

- How are a family doctor and her patient to set priorities – to choose which tasks need to be completed during this consultation and which can be left? Models that offer a comprehensive and detailed insight into the consulting process have limited applicability as a benchmark against which every single consultation should be assessed. In day-to-day consulting, choices have to be made about what to do and what to leave out. When is a consultation good enough? How do you know when to stop?
- There are things which go on during a family medicine consultation that do not appear on any of the lists of tasks in the established models. Does this mean that all family doctors are doing it wrong, or do the existing consultation models offer an incomplete view of what is happening? For example, the personality of the consulting family doctor has a considerable influence on how the consultation progresses.[15] What is the scope for personal variation between family doctors? Could a family doctor's fuller appreciation of her own personality be actively used to improve consultations?
- A task-based consulting model is inevitably stronger on the 'what' than on the 'how', so it will tell you what to do without telling you how to do it. How might tasks be translated into appropriate behaviours?
- What is in it for the family doctor? Is improved consulting performance consistent with more satisfaction for the consulter? If consultations in family practice are genuinely to become more co-operative and collaborative, is it too much to ask that both sides of the consultation might benefit? There is always the satisfaction of a job well done, but producing ever longer lists of 'tasks' risks just the opposite. Family doctors are known to be psychologically vulnerable,[6] and not good at coping with failure or criticism.[16] If there are more tasks to be done then a family doctor must take more time and be more dedicated. The family doctor may come to believe that the only answer is more self-sacrifice and more self-abasement. How is this likely to affect a group of people who are psychologically characterised by compulsive and perfectionist traits?[6]

John's first job as a family doctor was not going too well. He had deliberately chosen a salaried post working less than full-time because he wanted to concentrate on getting his clinical skills up to standard, and he did not want to feel exhausted all the time.

What he had not expected was that the patients he saw would be different from the ones he was used to. Many had long-standing problems which had defied the efforts of other family doctors, and they wanted to go through their symptoms in meticulous detail. Some expressed their disappointment at the treatment they had received so far, and John was not sure how he should respond to such criticism. Some patients brought long lists of things they wanted to talk about and seemed oblivious to the fact that other patients were waiting.

John despaired of ever being able to keep the customers satisfied while preserving his own sanity. He realised that for as long as he could remember he had been trying to do what other people wanted him to do. It had started with his parents. Then his teachers told him that to pass science exams one has to learn established facts and not think for oneself. Education by humiliation at medical school had almost reduced him to tears on occasion because his best was never quite good enough. Now John felt that the patients were trying to make him responsible for their problems.

- The consultation *stakeholders* are those people or groups who are affected by and so have a legitimate interest in what goes on in a family practice consultation. The patient is obviously the most important stakeholder, and the family doctor is equally clearly affected. Indeed in at least one respect the family doctor is affected more, since she will spend more time consulting than will an individual patient. The community of family doctors is also concerned about what happens, as the good name of the profession has to be upheld. The patient's family, carers and friends are stakeholders. The family practice has organisational needs. Other patients of the family practice, and society at large, are quite entitled to have some say in how the money is spent. And then there are always the lawyers. How can all of these possibly competing interests be juggled?
- Both training and experience produce demonstrable improvements in the consulting skills displayed by family doctors. To achieve an 'expert' perform-ance, a family doctor must be able to adapt her approach to her patient's needs, which requires a high degree of self-awareness, and also an awareness of the sort of patient that is being consulted with (P Worrall, personal communi-cation). Can this sort of sensitivity and awareness be actively learned? And does this mean that the kind of qualities that are usually associated with experience can be improved by training?

Taking advice

Family doctors offer their patients a highly complex and technical service. The technical quality of the service delivered is not likely to be fully appreciated by the recipients of the service. At the same time, the satisfaction (or dissatisfaction) of the recipients of the service affects the outcome.[9] It is the perennial expert's dilemma – how can patients be happy with a family doctor's performance when they probably do not fully understand what there is to be happy about?

Other professional groups in society face exactly the same problems, and in many cases are further along the path to finding solutions to those problems. Consumerism challenges the idea that the expert knows best. Money has become a universal exchange medium for both products and services, and people want to know what they are getting for their hard-earned cash. In businesses where the commercial imperative is particularly obvious, difficult lessons have had to be learned. It is appropriate that family doctors look at how others have managed their problems, in order to see what can be applied to their own situation.

The knowledge and experience of other professional groups are already being used in the development of medical practice. For instance, much of the research basis of the MRCGP video performance criteria derives from the work of psychologists, sociologists and anthropologists. Family doctors do not have a monopoly on the truth.

Looked at another way, it would be wrong to think that either family doctors or patients in a consultation completely ignore the experiences and influences of the rest of their existence. Taking one's car to be mended is in many respects like taking one's body to be healed. There are some singular differences as well, but to patients both must seem like submitting oneself to a closed expert world where the available information is only partially understood, where the potential costs are enormous, and where nearly all clients are left with the slight feeling that they have been 'ripped off'. The quality of customer service achieved by other professions that do an expert job is often higher than that offered by primary care. These are the service levels that our patients have come to expect, so it makes sense to look at and learn from the way in which our professional colleagues have dealt with the types of problem that primary care faces now.

Role, behaviour and acting

The role of a family doctor is the set of values, norms and beliefs that motivate her professional behaviour and actions. It provides the background from which all professional aspirations emerge, and as such it affects every consultation with every patient. A family doctor should be as clear as possible in her own mind about what her professional role is.

Reaching a decision about your professional role has two uses. It prompts some detailed thought about beliefs and values. It also provides a benchmark against which performance can be judged – if you don't know where you are going, then how do you know in which direction to travel and how will you know when you have arrived?

The role of a family doctor has both collective and personal dimensions. The collective dimension is the one shared with other family doctors, the aspects of the role that characterise the group of 'family doctors'. The personal dimension consists of the aspects of the role which mark out that family doctor as an individual, and which help her to make her unique contribution to patient care.

Thus each family doctor will have a slightly different idea about what her role is, and this does not matter so long as the role brings about behaviour which in general conforms to 'what family doctors do'. You would not expect a single-handed rural practitioner near retirement to have the same ideas about her role as a salaried family doctor just starting out in a large inner-city group practice. Perceptions of role will alter and evolve over time, and it is appropriate for the conscientious practitioner to be involved in a constant process of redefinition and refinement as far as her role is concerned.

Having decided what role she wishes to adopt, each family doctor must then work out how she is to portray it. Over time a battery of behaviours is used to express the role, and these behaviours will be different for different family doctors. Indeed it will often be necessary for each family doctor to have several different behaviours to express each aspect of her role. As communication is all to do with what is received, one can never be sure that a piece of behaviour will be interpreted as intended, so alternatives will have to be ready for use. Different patients may well need different approaches.

It would be unlikely that an individual patient would be exposed to all the aspects of their family doctor's chosen professional role, or to her full repertoire of professional behaviours. Different aspects of the role, each resulting in a package of behaviours, will be offered according to whatever seems appropriate to meet a patient need. A family doctor will select parts of her family doctor role to employ to best effect.

Actors are particularly good at working out a role, and at translating that role into elements of behaviour, using techniques that have stood the test of time. Of course some actors are better ('more convincing') than others, but then so are some family doctors more effective than others. The use of acting techniques in family medicine is not new. There already exists considerable experience in the use of actors in medical education and assessment, and acting skills are being actively promoted among doctors and medical students in order to develop a fuller appreciation of patient feelings.

Acting theory can also offer insight into the consulting process because in many respects a consultation is like a theatrical performance. People (patients to a family doctor, the audience to an actor) choose to pay a visit to a premises designed for and dedicated to the task (surgery, theatre) in order to receive a service (healthcare, entertainment) from someone specially trained to do the job (family doctor, actor).

Acting theory suggests that a theatrical performance can be looked at in the same way as the process by which changes occur in society as a whole.[17] In his book *The Rites of Passage*, published in 1908, Arnold van Gannep described three phases of social change.[18]

1. *Separation.* There is some sort of disruption to the established order of things, and those who are experiencing the disruption know that something is wrong or could be better, so they want to change it. To a potential patient, this is the stage when anxiety about a symptom reaches the point of wanting something done about it, leading up to the decision to consult. To a member of the audience, this is the decision to attend a performance – the wish to be entertained.
2. *Transition.* As far as those who want a change are concerned, clearly what has gone before does not work or is no longer working, or the initial disruption would not have occurred. Change is in order. During transition, people who want a change will critically evaluate almost any option, even those options which in normal times would be unthinkable. They are very receptive to new ideas even if those ideas violate established norms and values, such as the perception of what is 'proper' or 'nice'. All sorts of ideas are thrown into the arena for consideration – a process which might in another context be called 'brainstorming'   on the understanding that most of the ideas are either impractical, inappropriate or just plain wrong. To a patient (for, having decided to consult, this is what he now is) this is the consultation(s) during

which information is shared and processed, and management options are generated. To an actor, this is the actual performance.[1.1]

In order to cope with such apparent disorder, and involvement with often unwelcome information and hypotheses, participants in transition have to feel safe. Coping is assisted by the reassurance that the environment is recognised as a safe place for transition to occur. Clearly this has implications for surgery design and use.

3. *Reincorporation*. In this final phase, either the original disruption comes to be accepted, or an adjustment has occurred. A change has occurred in beliefs, knowledge and expectations, and the world will never be quite the same again. In the theatre, this is when the audience leaves. Patients, even when they are restored to complete health, will have the memory of what has occurred and any treatments required, and will have experiences of the organisation and individuals involved in their illness. They must be left fit to face the real world outside, the world of order and familiarity. The chaos of irregular thoughts and feelings must, as far as possible, be left behind with the performance.

The work of actors has more in common with that of family doctors than is at first apparent. Each must be clear about their role, and each must endeavour to portray their role to maximum effect. Each works in an environment that is both appropriate to the job and seen as appropriate for the job. And each deals with people when they are disorientated, suggestible and vulnerable.

The structure of the book

This book suggests a step-by-step guide to improving your consultations with patients and your own well-being. It is a re-evaluation of the available research and literature in the light of experience. The content of the book does not represent a comprehensive review of consulting skills and theories, and it is not an assessment tool. However, it does seek to address some of the practical problems that a consulting family doctor faces.

The role of a family doctor

The chapter on role explores in more detail the collective and personal dimensions of a family doctor's role. It discusses the relationship between role and behaviour. Suggestions are made about the parameters with which the behaviour produced by the role must comply. A series of seven questions, derived from acting theory, is offered as a system by which a family doctor can begin to consider the details of her own professional role.

[1.1] During a theatrical performance it may be thought necessary to remind the audience that normality is temporarily suspended, to emphasise the fact that in terms of ideas 'anything goes'. The performance may be punctuated by unexpected and inappropriate playfulness, silliness and gasp-inducing feats of prestidigitation. Is it stretching the analogy beyond breaking point to observe a parallel in the family doctor who performs a clinical examination or uses a piece of diagnostic equipment, even though she knows that in many cases such activity is unlikely to help in patient management?

'B' is for behaviour

The behaviour used in a consultation is the practical expression of a family doctor's role or motivations. However, consulting behaviour is only effective if it brings about the desired result. BARD is a practical approach to consulting, and the chapter on behaviour makes a number of suggestions about the 'how' of consulting to go alongside the 'what' of other consulting models.

'A' is for aims

Aims are the directions along which a family doctor wants to progress a consultation or a series of consultations. The chapter starts with some reasons why 'aims' are more appropriate than 'targets' in the family medicine consultation. The stakeholders to a consultation may have differing aims, and all deserve consideration. The number of things that might be done in every consultation is very large, and trying to do too much in each consultation does neither the patient nor the family doctor any good. A method for judging when a consultation is 'good enough' is discussed. BARD extends the taxonomy of consulting aims in a practical and realistic way.

'R' is for room

The spaces within which consultations are held – whether they be consulting rooms, clinics, patient houses, hospitals or even the local supermarket – have an impact on how well the consultations work. Some thought must be given to the effect of the spaces that are being used, and the adjustment of consulting skills needed to cope with this. How do you move around and use the spaces during a consultation? How should you dress for a consultation?

'D' is for dialogue

What words do you choose to use? Is jargon ever justified? What do patients want to hear? Are medical words helpful? How do you deal with accents and regional words? What strategies can be used to ensure that you and your patient are talking the same language? How should your speech be structured? Can your patients hear you? A family doctor's voice is a major consultation tool. How can it be used to maximum effect? All this and more is covered in the chapter on dialogue.

Training for BARD

The chapter on training is a series of suggested exercises designed to help the reader to increase their BARD competence. The exercises are derived partly from acting training and partly from experience with family doctors in training.

The ethics of BARD

Many readers will quite rightly have reservations about the use of acting techniques in order to pursue aims in a consultation, due to concern that this could be a deceitful and manipulative process. As might be expected, actors do not see the ethics of their profession in this way.

Is BARD helpful?

BARD offers a realistic and practical insight into family doctor consulting, encompassing areas where other models fear to tread. Is such a contention justified?

BARD:

- prompts reflection on the fundamental values of family medicine
- prompts reflection on the unique interaction between a particular patient and a particular doctor at a particular time
- stresses how the family doctor's personality can be used in a positive way within a consultation
- recognises that the legitimate aims of consulting are not only the biomedical ones
- encourages the examination of the consultation from the perspective of how it is likely to appear to a patient
- offers new possibilities with regard to the ways in which consulting skills can be developed and matured
- makes transparent what real family doctors actually do in their job.

But how does BARD make consulting less stressful? Surely if the BARD criteria have to be fulfilled in addition to an existing consultation model, doesn't that place further demands on the poor beleaguered family doctor? Well, no.

- The BARD family doctor's chosen professional role is in accordance with her personality, beliefs and values. The BARD family doctor is playing to her strengths.
- It is legitimate to do what all family doctors actually do, namely to adjust behaviour in order to achieve an aim. BARD is guilt-free.
- It is all right not to complete all of the potential consultation aims at every consultation. In fact, it is not remotely possible to complete all of the potential aims of a consultation every time. The BARD benchmark is 'When is a consultation good enough?'.
- 'Aims' are more realistic, more evidence based and more practical than 'targets'. Aims may be defined for the present and often for future consultations as well – setting a partial agenda for a subsequent consultation(s) recognises the continuity of family medical practice. The aims can also be shared with your patient, so the great ethical principle of autonomy is upheld.
- The person of a family doctor is not the same as her professional role, and her professional role is not the same as her behaviour. A family doctor only has a responsibility to do her job properly, and this is not the same as taking the blame for the symptoms of her patients. She has no supernatural powers, and can only deal with the possible. To the BARD family doctor, criticism is not a challenge to her person, but rather it is an observation that the role or a behaviour could do with some refinement. The observable behaviour is simply

the manifestation of the aspect of the family doctor's role which happens to be on display at that time.
• Pride in a job well done is a positive feeling that we could all do with experiencing more often.

Summary

The consulting skills of family doctors have improved immeasurably within a relatively short space of time. Overcoming the challenges facing primary care will inevitably require further improvements in consulting skills in the future. The solutions that are found to these challenges must not make the mental health of family doctors any worse. The established models of the consultation offer an incomplete analysis of what actually occurs, and by their structure may make consulting more stressful. Family doctors would do well to look at how others, and particularly actors, have addressed problems similar to those facing primary care today.

Performing consultations is probably the most important thing that family doctors do, and it demands their most pressing attention. The BARD approach seeks to build on the professional responsibility of family doctors to use all of the consultation tools at their disposal to improve their performance. Family doctors are already a high class act. BARD is a contribution to the ongoing discussions and development of the consultation. It is to their credit that family doctors are involved in such discussions, and are not prepared to be complacent about their performance.

References

1. Coulter A (1999) Paternalism or partnership? *BMJ.* **319**: 719–20.
2. Byrne PS and Long BEL (1976) *Doctors Talking to Patients.* HMSO, London.
3. MORI (2004) *Trust In Doctors*; www.mori.com/polls/2004/bma.shtml. Accessed 14 April 2004.
4. Kmietowicz Z (2001) GMC steps up hearings to deal with rise in cases. *BMJ.* **323**: 129.
5. Goffman E (1990) *The Presentation of Self in Everyday Life.* Penguin, Harmondsworth.
6. Royal College of General Practitioners (2002) *Stress and General Practice.* RCGP Information Sheet No 22. Royal College of General Practitioners, London.
7. Kmietowicz Z (2001) Quarter of family doctors want to quit, BMA survey shows. *BMJ.* **323**: 887.
8. Pendleton D, Schofield T, Tate P *et al.* (1984) *The Consultation: an approach to teaching and learning.* Oxford University Press, Oxford.
9. Silverman J, Kurtz S and Draper J (2004) *Skills for Communicating with Patients* (2e). Radcliffe Publishing, Oxford.
10. Tate P (2002) *The Doctor's Communication Handbook.* Radcliffe Medical Press, Oxford.
11. Neighbour R (1987) *The Inner Consultation.* Petroc, Newbury.
12. Royal College of General Practitioners (2005) *Membership (MRCGP) Examination. Membership by assessment of performance (MAP): video assessment of consulting skills in 2005.* Royal College of General Practitioners, London.
13. Stott NCH and Davies RH (1979) The exceptional potential of each primary care consultation. *J R Coll Gen Pract.* **29**: 201–5.
14. Pereira Gray D (1998) Forty-seven minutes for the patient. *Br J Gen Pract.* **48**: 1816–7.
15. Smith R (2003) Thoughts for new medical students at a new medical school. *BMJ.* **327**: 1430–3.

16. Jain A and Ogden J (1999) General practitioners' experiences of patients' complaints: qualitative study. *BMJ.* **318**: 1596–9.
17. Carlson M (1996) *Performance: a critical introduction.* Routledge, London.
18. van Gannep A (1960) *The Rites of Passage* (trans. MB Vizedon and GL Caffee). Chicago University Press, Chicago.

MRCGP video performance criteria 2005

1. The doctor is seen to encourage the patient's contribution at appropriate points in the consultation.
2. The doctor is seen to respond to signals (cues) that lead to a deeper understanding of the problem. **Merit**
3. The doctor uses appropriate psychological and social information to place the complaint(s) in context.
4. The doctor explores the patient's health understanding.
5. The doctor obtains sufficient information to include or exclude likely relevant clinical conditions.
6. The physical/mental examination chosen is likely to confirm or disprove hypotheses that could reasonably have been formed *or* is designed to address a patient's concern.
7. The doctor appears to make a clinically appropriate working diagnosis.
8. The doctor explains the problem in appropriate language.
9. The doctor's explanation incorporates some or all of the patient's health beliefs. **Merit**
10. The doctor specifically seeks to confirm the patient's understanding of the diagnosis. **Merit**
11. The management plan (including any prescription) is appropriate for the working diagnosis, reflecting a good understanding of modern accepted medical practice.
12. The patient is given the opportunity to be involved in significant management decisions.
13. In prescribing the doctor takes steps to ensure concordance, by exploring and responding to the patient's understanding of the treatment. **Merit**
14. The doctor specifies the conditions and interval for follow-up or review.

Chapter 2

The role of a family doctor

Introduction

The role of a family doctor is the set of values, norms and beliefs that she tries to adhere to – the principles that motivate her professional behaviour and actions. It is her fundamental intellectual engine, and it affects every consultation. Considering how important and central this role is to their professional performance, it is surprising that many family doctors go through their career paying little attention to their role, and never being clear exactly what that role is. The role that a family doctor wishes to portray demands just as much attention as any other aspect of her professional growth and development. It is relatively fixed, but nevertheless alters with time, knowledge and experience. A family doctor's role must be subject to a constant process of examination, re-evaluation and refinement.

BARD is a practical approach to consulting. It emphasises that how things are done is just as important as knowing what to do. Yet the 'how' of a consultation must be preceded by the 'what'. Only when a family doctor is clear about what she is trying to achieve in a consultation is it possible to consider how it might be achieved.

The role of a family doctor has a collective dimension. This is the shared values and beliefs held by all family doctors, which characterise family doctors as a group. An individual family doctor has little immediate choice in such areas, as the agenda is set by her peers. Changes in the collective dimension of the family doctor role do occur, but they tend to be relatively slow because of the inertia of tradition, and because of the number of people whose values and beliefs would need to be altered. Values and beliefs that have been held over years tend to be deeply ingrained, and change can be fiercely resisted.

The role of a family doctor also has a personal dimension. Every family doctor will have an additional set of motivations which will determine what sort of family doctor she wishes to be. As long as this personal dimension of role is consistent with the collective dimension, then a family doctor can make whatever choices she wishes. Her choices will affect her consultations, and will be an expression of her own personality and her own beliefs and values.

An understanding of the collective dimension of the role of a family doctor requires sensitivity to the views of other family doctors, and also to the expectations and beliefs of the patients whom they treat. An understanding of the personal dimension of the role of a family doctor requires self-awareness and self-honesty.

The ways in which the role of a family doctor might be portrayed are the subject of the next four chapters. This chapter will examine the various components of the family doctor's role itself, with a view to helping the individual family doctor to make her own choices about her role. The chapter will first discuss some broader aspects of the family doctor's role and its implications. Later sections will deal with a method, drawn from the experience of actors, by which the family doctor can set about becoming clear about her personal professional role.

Role and behaviour

A role is an internal mental construct, a set of aspirations, but it can only finally be judged by its manifestations – by what behaviour it produces. The inter-relationship between role and behaviour is so close that there is inevitable overlap between them – the role motivates the behaviour, but the behaviour indicates what the role is. Sometimes the words 'role' and 'behaviour' are used inter-changeably, but this is unhelpful as a family doctor's role is based on her fundamental personal beliefs and values and so is relatively permanent, whereas behaviour should be sufficiently alterable and flexible to deal with the differing demands of the job.

A branch of sociology that has been championed by Erving Goffman[1] suggests that all human interactions can be viewed as the participants engaging in a performance, so that all people are playing a role at all times. Goffman based his views both on the work of others and on his own observations of a crofting community on Shetland. The participant puts on what Goffman called a 'front' of behaviour, which is intended to pursue an agenda for the interaction. Included in the agenda may be personal objectives and/or the objectives of any 'team' or group of which the participant is a member. In his writing, the medical profession is cited several times as an important team whose members are likely to pursue team objectives. Goffman also described medicine as a 'sacred' profession, its status being beyond criticism. How times have changed.

The audience to such a front in many respects colludes in the performance. They have expectations of what will happen in a given situation, a sort of memory shorthand so that every social interaction does not have to be assessed afresh. If the front offends expectation, then disruption to the interaction occurs. The physical circumstances of the interaction (the 'set' and 'props') similarly influence what happens.

In many cases, a front is used so regularly that it becomes internalised, and as a result the performer is unaware that it is a front at all. A 'sincere' front is deemed to be one where the agenda that is prompting the front is fully believed by the performer. A 'cynical' front is one where the performer is aware that there is a deliberate motive for the behaviour, even if that motive is entirely beneficent ('it's for your own good').[1]

Applying this analysis of interactions to a consultation in family practice emphasises that motivation and performance are different, although they are clearly related. A family doctor's role and behaviour can be examined separately, and changes and improvements can be achieved in both or either of them. If family doctors are playing out a role in their consultations, then Goffman's suggestions also imply that patients are similarly portraying a role. They also have agendas and fronts which they are playing out (e.g. 'Well he would say that, wouldn't he?'). The pursuit of an agenda does not ensure its achievement – some fronts will be performed more competently than others.

Goffman's analysis might also be criticised. His ideas will naturally raise objections about the honesty of a process in which the participants are using deliberate behaviour to further an often unrevealed agenda. These objections are understandable, but ultimately unfounded, as will be discussed in the chapter on ethics. It is difficult to see the value of the distinction between the virtuous-sounding 'sincere' front and the more pejorative-sounding 'cynical' front as far as a consultation is concerned. When an improvement in patient care can be achieved at the same time as a performance criterion is fulfilled, then so much the better.

> By their fruits ye shall know them.
> Matthew 7:20

The validity of a family doctor's role can only be judged by others through the behaviour that it produces. It is probably possible for a family doctor to consistently behave in ways that do not accord with her perception of her role, so that the link between behaviour and motivation is not inevitable. However, the cognitive dissonance involved would be considerable, and the rest of the world would not notice. So what would be the point?

Role and status

As will be argued in the next chapter, on behaviour, there will be situations in a consultation (perhaps in every consultation) when a family doctor must be willing and able to project the fact that she is relatively more important (i.e. has higher status) than her patient. Patients do not take seriously advice offered by someone whom they believe to be of low status.[2] If medical advice is to be adhered to, then a family doctor must be able to behave in a high-status way in consultation when the situation requires it.

Despite the feeling among many family doctors themselves that their status has declined in recent years, there remains ample evidence that patients and society as a whole still hold family doctors in high esteem, and are prepared to allow them the privileges necessary to do their job. Examples of such evidence include the following.

- Patients generally trust their family doctor to do her work properly, even when most patients do not understand what 'doing her work properly' actually means.[3]
- Medical professionalism is the benchmark to which many other professions aspire.
- Family doctors are permitted a long and intensive education during which they make only a limited contribution to the community. Once educated, they keep their academic qualifications for life, but are under no obligation to use their knowledge and skills for the good of the society that has allowed their acquisition. Even though such an allowance is also made for other kinds of educational attainment, the sheer length of a family doctor's education makes the privilege more apparent.
- People are, in the main, prepared to pay family doctors rather more than an average worker for what they do. This is not an inevitable privilege. For example, in the former Soviet Union doctors were not considered to be as important as coal miners, and so were paid less.

- Family doctors are allowed to ask their patients for information which would never normally be released except perhaps to the closest of friends and family members. A patient is considered to be failing in his duty if he does not answer all of a family doctor's questions honestly.
- Family doctors are allowed into people's territory – their homes and bedrooms – often when there has been no previous acquaintance.
- Family doctors are entrusted with authorities by their patients:[4]
  - *sapiential authority* – family doctors know lots of things, and more than their patients
  - *moral authority* – family doctors are good people and deserve respect
  - *charismatic authority* – family doctors are important because they deal with difficult things, with life and death issues
  - *bureaucratic authority* – in the UK at least, family doctors are the main way of gaining access to medicines, hospitals, operations and financial sickness benefits.

The high regard in which society generally holds its family doctors should be used but not abused. It is legitimate to assume high status, and to behave in a high-status way, as long as this is likely to result in a better patient outcome. However, outside of this professional context it would be inappropriate and unethical to behave in such a way.

Role and obligation

A family doctor must feel comfortable in the social position that she has, since that position is an integral part of the consultation process. However, she must also be aware of the responsibilities and obligations that her position confers. If her role does not enable her to behave in the way that family doctors are supposed to, then she cannot expect to be given the privileges and authority accorded to all family doctors. She must be seen to deserve her position. She must also be clear that her authority is confined to the consulting room – the fact that a family doctor is good at consulting does not necessarily mean that she is good at other things.

Society is, of course, composed of individuals, and it is individuals with whom a family doctor interacts when consulting. As well as fulfilling her professional obligations to society at large, the family doctor must also be aware that different patients may have different ideas and expectations about how a family doctor should behave.

The obligations of the family doctor's role can be considered under four headings, namely efficacy, professionalism, patient expectations and personality, and every family doctor's chosen role must be consistent with these obligations. Each of the four headings encompasses patient-centred and doctor-centred aspects – an agreement to consult is based on the co-operation of the participants.

Efficacy

The role that a family doctor adopts must allow her to get the medicine right. This is an area that is under active promotion by family doctors as a group and also by governments and others on behalf of patients. There are many clinical guidelines to refer to, so ideas about what represents good practice are not hard to find. Patients deserve a family doctor who keeps herself up to date. Identifying and dealing with areas of ignorance is an important part of the process by which a family doctor can achieve continuous improvement.

Getting the medicine right means prescribing the right drugs and referring the right cases, but there are other considerations as well.

- The best person to deliver a particular element of care may well not be a family doctor but a different healthcare worker, and patients can reasonably expect to be treated by the person who is best able to deliver the treatment. A family doctor must not assume that she is the most competent person for every job in primary care.
- Dealing only with physical problems is not enough. Unless the psychological and social aspects of a patient's problems are also addressed then overall the treatment is sub-standard.
- Efforts should be made to secure patient satisfaction and empowerment, because this results in better adherence to treatments and better outcomes.[5]

Professionalism

The role that a family doctor adopts must allow her to behave in a professional manner. Professionals adhere to a vocation or calling which requires prolonged education in an institution of higher learning or a hospital.[6] Most people do not undergo such an education, and so take it on trust that a professional will do her job properly and apply her area of expertise in a competent manner for the benefit of others. It is a characteristic of a professional group that people have trust in its members, and (conversely) professional status is accorded by society to those groups whose ability to do their job properly is a matter of trust. For all its aura of quaintness, trust in a family doctor remains an important part of the relationship that she has with her patients, and so is an essential aspect of the care process.[7]

A family doctor who behaves in an unprofessional way, or in a way that is radically different from the behaviour of the generality of family doctors, may be regarded as a threat to the good name of all family doctors. Professional trust takes a long time to establish, and as this trust is integral to the care process, behaviour which might compromise the trust that people have in their family doctors is not something to be undertaken lightly. This is not to say that things can never change, or that there is never any justification for radically different behaviour. A professional should constantly seek to improve her performance. Each new generation of family doctors quite rightly wants to improve on what has gone before, and each family doctor wants to 'do her own thing'. The maintenance of enthusiasm requires a healthy scepticism about tradition, a sense that things could and ought to be done better. Yet a family doctor who wants to change the relationships that she has with her patients must at the same time have due regard to her professional status and take care not to betray the trust that her patients have in her.

Patient expectations

The role that a family doctor adopts must take account of the expectations that her patients are likely to have of her. Society at large has expectations of how family doctors should behave, not just in their professional role but also in their private lives. As a pillar of society, a family doctor will want to avoid scandal. Behaviour may be noticed not because the behaviour itself is remarkable – newsworthiness depends not just on the behaviour itself but also on who is doing it.

> It was a snowy, sludgy evening during which John had skidded into the car in front and broken a headlight. Later on, after a couple of beers, he was pulled over by the police because of the damaged light, and was breath-alysed as a matter of routine. Although the test was well within the limit for safe driving, the officer made several remarks about such behaviour from '*a man in your position.*'

Patients who attend their family doctor regularly will also have developed specific expectations based on their ongoing relations with that one family doctor, and so may be more tolerant of idiosyncrasy. In general, however, patients want a family doctor who sounds, looks and behaves like a family doctor.

> Sometimes John got quite fed up with the stories that patients would tell him, often repeatedly, about a doctor – now retired from the family practice – who developed a reputation as a 'character'. John remembered him as a bad-tempered and difficult man. What patients remembered was his occasional habit of offering them cigarettes and whisky during consulta-tions. John was not at all sure that this promoted the good name of family doctors, even if it delighted the patients involved.

Personality

The role adopted by a family doctor must take account of her own personality. Most family doctors want to express themselves, and that includes the expression of their personality, through their work. Many have entered family practice specifically because they want the freedom to behave as they think best, without outside constraints. The family doctor's personality may well be the reason why she ended up in the job in the first place.

A family doctor's personality is probably her most powerful therapeutic tool in consultations.[8] It is one of the attributes that confers a uniqueness on each interaction between an individual patient and an individual family doctor. Even if she tried to behave in a way that was at variance with her personality, there is a limit to the degree and frequency with which a family doctor can cause her behaviour to deviate from her natural traits and inclinations. A major strength of family medicine is the way in which family doctors express their personality through their work.

Role and a job description

A family doctor's role and her behaviour are closely linked. Her perception of her professional role motivates her behaviour, and her role can also be implied from her observed behaviour. Accordingly, having a job description for a family doctor goes some way towards suggesting a role for that family doctor.

A job description for a family doctor also has implications for the training, assessment and discipline of family doctors. In addition, once a description of what a family doctor does has been drawn up, it also assumes a moral power – this is what family doctors are supposed to do, this is what patients (and others) can expect from a family doctor, this is what patients are entitled to, and so on.

There was an early attempt to describe what a family doctor does in 1972 with the publication by the Royal College of General Practitioners (RCGP) of *The Future General Practitioner*.[9] The text of this can be found in Appendix 2.1. This is not a detailed job description, and the specifics mentioned mainly deal with the issues that British family doctors were wrestling with at the time, namely adequate premises, working in teams, and framing a diagnosis in physical, psychological and social terms. Not much, then, about what patients can expect, how family doctors should be trained, or the ongoing development of the profession. The definition cannot be described as a comprehensive outline of how a modern family doctor fills her working time, even though it does have the advantage of brevity.

The services that a family doctor undertakes to provide for her patients represent another form of job description. For instance, the *Terms of Service for Doctors in General Practice*,[10] which all UK family doctors signed up to in 1989, and the *New GMS Contract*,[11] adopted in 2003, both give a comprehensive list of the services that family doctors should provide for their patients. This might be termed the 'John Wayne' approach – a family doctor's job is to deliver the services that family doctors deliver, or 'a family doctor's got to do what a family doctor's got to do'.

Another (and by some way the most comprehensive) example of a job description for a family doctor was endorsed by the World Organisation of National Colleges, Academies and Academic Associations of General Practitioners/Family Physicians (WONCA) Europe Region in June 2002[12] (*see* Appendix 2.2). It is hard to disagree with anything contained in this definition. It is a more wide-ranging and comprehensive description of the underlying principles of family medicine, and as such represents more of a development on *The Future General Practitioner* than the *New GMS Contract*.

Does role awareness help?

A family doctor who is more conscious of her role and its implications is in a better position to portray her role to the best advantage for her patients. A family doctor who is clear in her mind (with reasons) about what she can and cannot do, and perhaps more particularly about what she will and will not do, is able to offer a consistent and realistic service. It does her patients no good at all when a family doctor makes promises that she cannot keep. On the other hand, clarity of role should lead to reliability of behaviour – a promise that is likely to be kept.

Equally compelling is the probability that role awareness will also benefit the doctor herself. Accepting the idea that a family doctor is permitted to derive benefit from her consulting may seem a little radical when family doctors are characterised by devotion and selflessness, but as a family doctor will spend much of her professional life consulting with patients, drawing a positive rather than a negative effect from each consultation is a significant advantage.

The context of the job of a family doctor brings inevitable stresses. For instance, medicine by its nature deals with pain and death, so that people usually consult a family doctor when there is something wrong rather than when all is going well. Thus there is a clear danger that a family doctor who takes her patients' problems personally will feel perpetually guilty.

At present the mental health of family doctors is not very good.

- Family doctors tend to take criticism badly.[13]
- The suicide rate among male family doctors is significantly above average, and the suicide rate among female family doctors in the UK is twice the national population average.[14]
- Female family doctors have a tendency towards perfectionism, a trait that predisposes to depression.[14]

Any way of reducing the work stress and so preventing the mental ill health of a family doctor is to be welcomed. Role awareness is one way of relieving work stress.

- Using Goffman's analysis,[1] a role can be criticised without criticising the person who is portraying it. Similarly, the way in which the role is translated into a behaviour or 'front' is equally eligible for scrutiny. The person is not the same as the role, and the role is not the same as the behaviour. There can be a scientific detachment which enables training and improvements to be made without the individual being subjected to personal attack. Evidence for the benefit of such an approach can be found in the literature on negotiation ('separate the problem from the personality'[15]), and in the technique of *cognitive reframing* in psychological therapies.[16]
- A family doctor is allowed to derive satisfaction from her work. The role that she has chosen is consistent with her collective and personal professional principles, so playing out the role can be accompanied by a sense of satisfaction. Both the family doctor and the patient are benefiting from a truly collaborative and mutually supportive interaction. A family doctor who is doing the things that she believes in can enjoy the opposite of cognitive dissonance – or what the psychologist Leon Festinger referred to as *cognitive consonance*.
- Role awareness includes being aware of the role of others. For an individual patient this might be termed the 'hidden agenda'. An angry patient is probably angry with everyone, and not just with his family doctor. Managers are compelled by their calling to promote the latest targets, especially if they are eligible for a performance bonus. Being aware that others are playing a role makes interactions less perplexing and stressful.

Choosing a role

So far this chapter has offered some general thoughts about how an individual family doctor might start to think about the professional role that she wishes to portray. This section will suggest a method, using a series of questions that you can ask yourself, of looking at more specific areas of a family doctor's professional role, and in particular the personal dimension of your professional role. Reflecting on the questions should provide a sound basis for fuller role awareness. The method is adapted from a technique that is well established in the training of actors, who are after all experts in developing and portraying a role.

The seven questions

Some lucky people maintain throughout their lives a crystal clear idea of what kind of person they want to be and therefore how they should behave towards the rest of the world. Others, probably the majority, spend their time fumbling through a mire of competing considerations and feelings, never having a proper idea of what they are trying to do, and consequently never having the satisfaction of achieving their objectives.

Stanislavsky was the professional name of Konstantin Sergeivich Alexeyev. Born in Moscow in 1865, he joined the Moscow Arts Theatre in 1898 and there developed his ideas on acting, which came to be known as 'the method'. When he was forced to give up acting himself because of poor health, he continued to teach and write. Although he died in 1938, his books are still in print and remain essential reading for students of the theatre.

Stanislavsky suggested that an actor could develop a theatrical role by answering a set of questions. There were originally either nine or ten questions (depending on the source).[17] Here the number of suggested questions has been reduced to seven, and they have been adapted for use by a family doctor.

Question 1   Who am I? What are my principles?

This is an invitation for the family doctor to reflect on her norms, values and beliefs – the basic principles that she tries to adhere to in her professional work – at a very fundamental level. At this level, the principles that are applied in her professional context will be a subset of those that she applies to her whole life. For example, if a family doctor believes in fairness and justice, this will be reflected in her personal life as well as in her professional role. Religious and political beliefs may well contribute to the principles that are held.

Principles that are held at this level can usually be expressed in terms of single words or short phrases, such as 'fairness', 'justice', 'consideration for others' and 'sanctity of life'. A suitable question to ask yourself might be 'What sort of family doctor do I want to be?'. Principles do not have to be invented – they already exist, but frequently in a muddled and unsorted form. Time spent on reflection will identify what the principles are, make them explicit, and so make them available for analysis.

Although they are a subset of her overall life principles, a family doctor's professional principles are inevitably distinct. For instance, all parents worry about their children, whether they are family doctors or not. This is a state of all-pervading concern entirely appropriate to those who are raising children. However, the same level of anxiety is not appropriate for a family doctor who is treating a sick child. It is impracticable for a family doctor to worry day in, day out about her young patients – a management decision is made and implemented, and the family doctor moves on to the next case. This is one reason why doctors of all kinds have such difficulty giving proper medical treatment to members of their own family – the relationship is not a doctor–patient relationship, so the normal rules of consultation and decision making do not work.

There is no 'correct' set of professional principles for a family doctor. As all family doctors have different personalities, their norms, values and beliefs will also be different, and principles that do not fit with the family doctor's personality are unlikely to be sustainable. Some of the principles that are held by a family doctor will be readily accepted by all family doctors, and this is the collective dimension of a family doctor's role. However, there is in addition the personal dimension of her role.

As well as having slightly different principles, individual family doctors will want to emphasise different aspects of their role. Some aspects of the chosen role will be ones that the family doctor wants to portray at all times, and others will be 'optional extras' to be fitted into consultations as the need arises. Some family doctors will want to emphasise their professionalism, while others will consider their obligations as a public servant to be more important. Some are scientists ever on the lookout for interesting cases, while others see primary care as a branch of the social and welfare care services.

Having completed his training, John felt that he had a pretty clear idea of what his patients and professional colleagues expected of him, and was happy to play out that role. At the same time, he felt that he had something extra to bring to the job. He wanted in particular to make sure that all of his patients, especially the deprived ones, received the best care he could deliver, and he wanted to be able to understand the working environments of his patients. After a couple of beers he liked to think of himself as a 'people's doctor.'

Question 2   What has happened in my life to develop my principles?

Some personality traits, especially those that predispose to depression and work stress, are over-represented in medical students.[14] Presumably such traits are the result of heredity and early life. For example, entrants to UK medical schools are mainly drawn from a relatively narrow section of society.[18] Such a middle-class background will tend to promote middle-class values. In addition, all family doctors will have successfully undergone a prolonged education, an experience that will not have been shared by many of their patients.

The people who may have influenced a family doctor's principles include parents, teachers, other students, work colleagues and trainers, as well as any other influential people (e.g. priests or sports coaches) incidentally encountered through life. Many family doctors will be able to recall their 'heroes' – those who have left a good impression either as people or as doctors (or both), and whom the family doctor would like to emulate. The principles held by such heroes (or what the family doctor assumes those principles to have been) will inevitably have a lasting effect.

> When John started training future family doctors himself, he found that he repeatedly remembered and quoted his own trainer from many years before. His trainer was from an aristocratic family, and had sent his children to private schools, something that John could never agree with. However, John's old trainer just oozed calmness, confidence and competence, was a highly effective clinician, and attracted the almost universal affection of his patients. It made John realise the responsibilities that being in a training position involved, and he was always aware of the kind of impression he was having on his own trainees.

> **Question 3** What order of priority do I give to my principles?

As well as identifying what her principles are, a family doctor must also decide which of those principles are more important and which are less important to her. Not all principles will be equally firmly held. A list of principles should look a bit like a list of 'good things about humanity'. All of them are important, and no one likes to think that they are not sticking to their principles. However, the job of a family doctor requires compromises, so that a less important principle sometimes has to be dropped in favour of a more important one. Once a principle has been overridden, it is easier to override it again, and sometimes it risks being permanently abandoned. This would be a mistake, as it is quite depressing for a family doctor to feel that her principles are disappearing one by one. It is better to hang on to the principle, but to accept that there are times and circumstances when other things take priority.

One way of assessing the strength with which a belief or a value is held is to use a Likert scale, named after the American educator and organisational psychologist Rensis Likert (1903–81), who worked extensively on management theory. Present the belief as a statement, and then respond on a five-point scale. A suitable example might be:

A family doctor should always be honest with her patients.

The range of allowed responses is as follows:

- strongly agree
- agree
- neither agree nor disagree
- disagree
- strongly disagree.

A more flexible approach would be to use two opposing statements and place them at opposite ends of a line. You would then mark on the line where you think your own attitudes lie. For example:

In a consultation in primary care:

The rights of the   The rights of the
patient are paramount – – – – – – – – – – – – – – doctor are paramount

The relative priorities of different principles will vary according to the circumstances.

- 'Consideration for others' and 'sanctity of life' probably figure on most family doctors' lists of principles. But which of these is more important when dealing with a request for a termination of pregnancy? Is it the right to life of the fetus, or the rights of the woman to control her own life? The relative priorities given to these two principles will affect whether a family doctor is inclined to support or block the termination request.
- When a patient first presents with diabetes, they have a new set of symptoms which are disorganised, uncontrolled and probably frightening. At this stage what is needed is a family doctor who is prepared to step in and take over some of the load of anxiety, to act in a reassuring and confident way to get things on track. Later, when a diagnosis has been made and a plan implemented, the time is right to talk about smoking and exercise, and to re-establish patient autonomy and responsibility. Like the best jokes or soufflés, a consultation can fail if the timing is wrong.

> In his professional life, John tried at all times to understand the viewpoint of his patients and to empathise with their troubles. During a consultation with a very upset middle-aged woman, this patient told John that the reason she was so distressed was because her son had decided to marry a black woman. On John's list of fundamental values, 'non-racist' rated as high as 'empathy' and 'professional'. John was relieved when the patient decided not to return for her follow-up appointment.

Question 4   What are my inner characteristics?

Different people think in different ways. Being aware of her own thinking preferences enables a family doctor to play to her mental strengths, and to identify areas where she may have to make a special effort. It also allows her to understand that the thinking preferences of other people may well be different from her own, and to compensate accordingly.

For example, people have different preferences concerning how they deal with other people and information. The Myers–Briggs Type Indicator (MBTI)[19] identi-fies four sets of opposing pairs of cognitive features and, depending on which feature of each pair a person tends towards, it thereby distinguishes 16 types of people. The four pairs of features can be summarised as follows.

1. *Extroversion* and *Introversion* (E and I). People who prefer Extroversion tend to focus on the outer world of people and things. People who prefer Introversion tend to focus on the inner world of ideas and impressions.
2. *Sensing* and *Intuition* (S and N [iNtuition]). People who prefer Sensing tend to focus on the present and on concrete information (evidence) gained from their senses. People who prefer Intuition tend to focus on the future, with a view towards patterns and possibilities.
3. *Thinking* and *Feeling* (T and F). People who prefer Thinking tend to base their decisions on logic and on objective analysis of cause and effect. People who prefer Feeling tend to base their decisions primarily on values and on subjective evaluation of person-centred concerns.
4. *Judgement* and *Perception* (J and P). People who prefer Judgement tend to like a planned and organised approach to life and prefer to have things settled. People who prefer Perception tend to like a flexible and spontaneous approach to life and prefer to keep their options open.

Considerable research has been done on the 16 types of people distinguished by these preferences, looking at their characteristics, their mental abilities, and the type of job they might do well. Research from America suggests that all MBTI groups are represented among doctors, but over the years there has been a reduction in Sensing with Perception preferences, and a trend towards an increase in Judging preference. Specialists in family care typically have a preference for Introversion and Feeling.[20]

A family doctor who so wishes can assess her MBTI using one of the published sets of questionnaires. There is also a close correlation between the results of formal testing and what a person thinks their results will be, having looked at the pairs of cognitive features.

The MBTI indicates thinking preferences. It does not suggest that a person is unable to think in any other way, just that it will feel a little unusual for him to do so, and he may not be very good at it due to lack of practice.

In general terms, doctors and their patients tend to have different MBTIs. This may be particularly important for communication in a consultation.[21]

> John wanted to portray his role as a family doctor in a way that fitted in with his natural tendencies. Once on a course he checked his MBTI and found that he was an ITNJ. He recognised that his preference was to be introverted because (for instance) he hated going to parties, but this was not a trait that he particularly welcomed, as the extroverts always seemed to be more impressive and having more fun. He also felt most comfortable in situations where doubt was at a minimum – when he was wrestling with a

Continued

high blood pressure rather than a social crisis. He knew that the job would often present challenges where these preferences would have to be over-ridden, so that he needed to deliberately work on forms of behaviour that would enable him to do this. He also realised that his tendency was to be thoughtful rather than up-front, and whereas he saw this as a feature of his introspectiveness, colleagues interpreted his behaviour as indicating hidden intellectual depths, which John was not sure was a justified assessment.

Question 5 What do my patients and work colleagues think of me?

This question attempts to assess how near or far away a family doctor feels she is from fulfilling her chosen role. A principle is usually a highly laudable objective, and modesty would prevent most family doctors from expressing the view that they always achieved their principles. Holding a principle is a type of wishful thinking. It would be a very poor principle that could be achieved without any effort. Indeed it might be argued that a principle, by its very nature, is unattainable, and adherence to a principle represents a commitment to a cause rather than a belief that the pursuit of a cause is ever adequately completed.

Making an honest appraisal (avoiding false modesty) of where she is now is a good way for a family doctor to assess where her priorities for the future lie. If she is missing one principle by a mile but is near to achieving another, then it makes sense to do work in the area of greatest shortfall.

Question 5 also encourages the family doctor to reflect on her relationships with her patients and colleagues, to see how near she is to proficiently presenting the role that she has chosen. In order to be valid, the conclusions of such reflection should be informed by evidence. Looking for deficiencies is always a rather anxiety-provoking exercise, which is why using evidence to reinforce an opinion is so important. Patients and colleagues may well be of the opinion that a family doctor is behaving in a principled way, even if she herself has her doubts about this. If a family doctor has repeatedly not lived up to her own hopes and expectations, clearly there is a problem. However, if (and this is much more likely) she manages to keep to her principles most of the time, but has an occasional lapse, then there is no cause for alarm.

John believed that if he could stay on good personal terms with his patients he would be in a win–win situation – he would feel better and his patients would feel better. Consequently he took it very badly when, for the first time, a patient made it very plain that she did not think much of him either as a person or as a family doctor. John brooded on this for the rest of the surgery, and made a point of telling the duty receptionist what had happened, ostensibly to see if there had been any moans or grumbles in the waiting room, but in reality to get some reassurance that his patient's view was not shared by others.

The duty receptionist told John that this patient had fallen out with many of the other family doctors and several other members of staff, and this made John feel a bit better. She also mentioned that John's surgeries were already booked up for the next week, and she pointed out that if everyone found him so unpleasant and incompetent then his surgeries would not be so well patronised.

Question 6 Where am I?

The emphasis that a family doctor will wish to place on different aspects of her role will depend on time, place and context.

Time

At different times in her career a family doctor will either want, or be required, to emphasise different aspects of her role. For example, a young or inexperienced family doctor may well want to expend most of her enthusiasm establishing a reputation among her patients and fellow workers for clinical competence, coping with the workload, reliability, and good communication and interpersonal relationships. At the same time she may want to demonstrate her powers of energy and innovation so that she can help the family practice to develop. On the other hand, she will not normally be overly involved in organisational issues, or be expected to exhibit the skills needed to deal with patients with whom she has had a relationship for many years, because in her case such patients do not yet exist.

An older family doctor will have a rather different role agenda. The aspects of her professional role that she will find necessary may include, for example, having a calming and steadying influence, offering support and advice when something happens that the younger family doctors in the practice have not had to deal with before, and coping with the ongoing and accumulating problems of an ageing patient cohort. Her generation would be expected to be running the show, and she must be aware that her opinion could make or break a new innovation in the practice. She may be invited to become involved in a wider political way on committees and other organisational bodies.

John had spent most of his professional career regarding himself as a young tyro, sniping against the established order of family medicine but not (in his own mind) taking on any responsibility for it. On his fiftieth birthday, while examining his grey hairs in the mirror, he realised that he was actually older than the Prime Minister. His generation was now in charge – of family practice and also of the country. If changes to his profession were needed, then it was up to him and his peers to get on and do something.

Place

A family doctor will need to emphasise different aspects of her role depending on the physical circumstances in which she is working. The demands of working in a deprived, inner-city area are not the same as those of working in an isolated rural community. An inner city family doctor will need to be able to offer the understanding and supporting aspects of her role to cope with her patients' expected requirements. Attention to acute interventional medicine or minor surgery may well be less important, because a secondary care centre is likely to be nearby. However, she may have to develop some specific skills – for instance, in the fields of child protection and drug abuse. A rural family doctor will certainly need some first aid skills. She may also, due to geographical and professional isolation, have more difficulty in keeping her clinical knowledge up to date. Her team may well be small, and this requires a different set of skills to those needed for working in a larger team.

Context

The team in which a family doctor works will have organisational needs, and she must expect to take her share of responsibility for these. If she is in a team that does not have any members with well-developed leadership skills, this is an aspect of her role that she will have to emphasise prominently. If the team already has a leader, then it may be clinical governance or personnel issues that need to be worked on. If, say, a family doctor feels that being on good terms with her co-workers is an important aspect of team development and healthcare delivery, and she finds that team relationships are poor, then she has a responsibility to do something about this even if displaying team-building skills does not come easily to her.

Question 7   What long-term effects do I want?

How do you see yourself doing your job in five, 10 or 20 years' time? The role that a family doctor chooses must be sustainable at least for the foreseeable future. It is never possible to predict the future with complete accuracy. The family doctor may change. Her patients may change. Almost certainly the social and organisational context within which she is working will change. The professional principles that have been adopted may be time limited. For example, a young doctor may wish to express her commitment to continuity of care by providing out-of-hours services to some or all of her patients while she is young and energetic, but understands that with advancing age she will probably be unable to maintain this level of commitment. Principles that have been adopted out of a sense of duty are also those that there may be a particular inclination to drop as soon as practicable, when the duty has been done and the family doctor feels that she has earned an honourable discharge.

   A family doctor who is pursuing distinct beliefs and values through her career will find that her efforts have momentum. Patients and team workers will get used to how she behaves and expect similar behaviour in future. A reputation will be developed. A family doctor who majors in empathy and understanding, and who believes in the social origins of anxiety and depression, should expect that word will get around among patients that she is good to talk to if you are fed up. As a consequence, patients with these kinds of problems will be over-represented in her surgeries, and will expect the time and consideration that the family doctor has given to others in the past. A family doctor who is engaged in large numbers of consultations where empathy and understanding are required will certainly have plenty of opportunities to fulfil her principles by expressing these aspects of her role, but may also feel that there is a limit to her capacity to cope. You can have too much – even of a good thing. The family doctor's professional survival may come more prominently on to the agenda, with a resulting rearrangement of role priorities.

A chosen professional role must be subjected to a continuing process of examination, review and refinement. Changes will invariably be needed, if not in the elements of the role (which by their nature are relatively fixed) then in the relative priority that is given to each element. The nature of such changes and the appropriate timing of the changes can both be difficult to get absolutely right. For example, a family doctor who is approaching retirement must be prepared to start disassembling the personal social ties that she has spent a professional lifetime building up, so that her patients can be successfully transferred over to the next generation of practitioners.

Mrs Large lived up to her name, and became one of John's regulars after his senior partner retired. After several frustrating consultations for vague symptoms that never seemed to quite fit into any physical or psychological diagnostic category, John was starting to despair about what to do next. Clearly neither a cure nor her changing doctor were on the agenda, so he spent a few minutes considering his dilemma and trying to work out an action plan that both he and Mrs Large could live with.

On reflection, it was apparent to John that his consultations with patients fell into three broad categories. Type 1 consultations were those with a strong physical content – puzzles which almost always had a 'right answer'. These were the heart attacks, the chest infections, the cases with clear diagnostic criteria and an obvious management plan. John felt that his undergraduate training had equipped him particularly for this type of consultation – quick, incisive and mutually satisfying.

Type 2 consultations were needed when there was a predominantly psychological component. The depressed patient needed guidance to see what was happening to them, and a firmness when suggesting a management plan which was slightly inconsistent with the 'patient autonomy' part of John's training in medical ethics. For the psychotics and addicts, a healthy scepticism about the accuracy of the patient's narrative was needed – patients with thought disorders could not be 'trusted' to tell the truth, and the real problem had to emerge from many different sources and from one-step-back observations of behaviour.

Consultations with Mrs Large never seemed to fit in the type 1 or type 2 categories, so John tried to think about times when things had gone either

Continued

well or badly, to put together a type 3 strategy. Mrs Large needed to be kept going until the next consultation, because there would always be a next consultation. First, type 3 consultations always took a long time, but once John realised that he was engaged in a type 3 he became more tolerant of over-running. Only a minority of patients needed type 3 consultations, and attempts not to run a type 3 with someone who needed one just caused frustration, as well as lasting just as long if not longer. Secondly, the technical medicine had to be right. John knew that frequent attenders are more likely to be ill, and in addition he wanted to be seen to be clinically competent by Mrs Large. Patients who needed a type 3 consultation had invariably been 'failed' by other doctors, and indeed stories of these failures were a regular part of type 3 consultations. For John this had what he felt sure was the intended effect of making him feel defensive. Therefore the third element of a type 3 consultation was to emphasise the co-operative dimension of the consultation, or – put another way – John was prepared to do whatever Mrs Large wanted him to do (within the bounds of reason and safety), so that she shared the responsibility for the next management failure. Fourthly, John wanted to emphasise the social element of their relationship, to try and build up Mrs Large's trust that he would do his best for her. He did this by spending a few seconds discussing her numerous grandchildren, and where possible sharing brief anecdotes about his own children.

Summary

The role of a family doctor has two dimensions. The collective dimension is motivated by a desire to show family doctors as a group in a particular light. The personal dimension is the way in which a particular family doctor wants to be viewed, according to her own principles. Choices about role are there to be made, particularly in the personal dimension which is unique for each family doctor. However, there are four over-arching considerations that must govern the role which a family doctor chooses, namely *efficacy, professionalism, patient expectations* and *personality*. Using a method derived from the training of actors, a further detailed insight may be gained to help the family doctor to decide what sort of family doctor she wants to be.

A family doctor who has a firm idea of her role – balancing all of the competing personal, professional and social considerations – is in a much better position to do her job to the best of her ability. She is likely to consult more effectively and to experience less work stress. The role provides a background against which the family doctor performs her job. The next four chapters discuss how the role can be translated into a performance. The aims and behaviour used in consulting, the way that the surgery is constructed and arranged, and the words used while consulting all depend on the role that the family doctor is trying to portray.

References

1. Goffman E (1990) *The Presentation of Self in Everyday Life*. Penguin, Harmondsworth.
2. Johnstone K (1981) *Impro*. Methuen, London.
3. MORI (2004) *Trust In Doctors*; www.mori.com/polls/2004/bma.shtml. Accessed 14 April 2004.
4. Pendleton D, Schofield T, Tate P *et al.* (1984) *The Consultation*. Oxford University Press, Oxford.
5. Silverman J, Kurtz S and Draper J (2004) *Skills for Communicating with Patients* (2e). Radcliffe Publishing, Oxford.
6. www.lactlaw.com. Accessed 9 July 2004.
7. Fugelli P (2001) Trust – in general practice. *Br J Gen Pract.* **51**: 575–9.
8. Smith R (2003) Thoughts for new medical students at a new medical school. *BMJ.* **327**: 1430–3.
9. Royal College of General Practitioners (1972) *The Future General Practitioner: learning and teaching*. Royal College of General Practitioners, London.
10. Department of Health (1989) *Terms of Service for Doctors in General Practice*. HMSO, London.
11. NHS Confederation and the British Medical Association (2003) *Investing in General Practice: new GMS contract*. NHS Confederation and the British Medical Association, London.
12. Allen J, Gay B, Crebolder H *et al.* (2002) The European definitions of the key features of the discipline of general practice: the role of the GP and core competencies. *Br J Gen Pract.* **52**: 526–7.
13. Jain A and Ogden J (1999) General practitioners' experiences of patients' complaints: qualitative study. *BMJ.* **318**: 1596–9.
14. Royal College of General Practitioners (2002) *Stress and General Practice*. RCGP Information Sheet No. 22. Royal College of General Practitioners, London.
15. Gourlay R (1987) *Negotiation for Managers*. Mercia Publications, London.
16. Goleman D (1996) *Emotional Intelligence*. Bloomsbury Publishing, London.
17. Jones E (1998) *Teach Yourself Acting*. Hodder Headline, London.
18. British Medical Association (2004) *Medicine Dominated by Highest Social Classes, BMA Report Shows*; www.bma.org.uk. Accessed 10 July 2004.
19. Briggs-Myers I and Myers P (1988) *Gifts Differing*. Oxford Psychologists Press, Oxford.
20. Stilwell NA, Wallick MM, Thal SE *et al.* (2000) Myers–Briggs type and medical specialty choice: a new look at an old question. *Teach Learn Med.* **12**: 14–20.
21. Clack GB, Allen J and Head JO (2004) Personality differences between doctors and their patients: implications for the teaching of communication skills. *Med Educ.* **38**: 177–86.

The Future General Practitioner, 1972[9]

The general practitioner is a doctor who provides personal, primary and continuing care to individuals and families. He may attend his patients in their homes, in his consulting room or sometimes in hospital. He accepts the responsibility for making an initial decision on every problem his patient may present to him, consulting with specialists when he thinks it appropriate to do so. He will usually work in a group with other general practitioners, from premises which are built or modified for the purpose, with the help of paramedical colleagues, adequate secretarial staff and all the equipment which is necessary. Even if he is in single-handed practice, he will work in a team and delegate when necessary. His diagnosis will be composed in physical, psychological and social terms. He will intervene educationally, preventively and therapeutically to promote his patient's health.

WONCA Europe, 2002[12]

General practice/family medicine is an academic and scientific discipline, with its own educational content, research, evidence base and clinical activity, and a clinical specialty orientated to primary care.

1. *The characteristics of the discipline of general practice/family medicine are that it:*
   (a) is normally the point of first medical contact within the healthcare system, providing open and unlimited access to its users, dealing with all health problems regardless of age, sex, or any other characteristic of the person concerned
   (b) makes efficient use of healthcare resources through co-ordinating care, working with other professionals in the primary care setting, and managing the interface with other specialties, taking an advocacy role for the patient when needed
   (c) develops a person-centred approach, orientated to the individual, his or her family and their community
   (d) has a unique consultation process, which establishes a relationship over time, through effective communication between doctor and patient
   (e) is responsible for the provision of longitudinal continuity of care as determined by the needs of the patient
   (f) has a specific decision-making process determined by the prevalence and incidence of illness in the community
   (g) manages simultaneously both acute and chronic health problems of individual patients
   (h) manages illness which presents in an undifferentiated way at an early stage in its development, which may require urgent intervention
   (i) promotes health and well-being by both appropriate and effective intervention
   (j) has specific responsibility for the health of the community
   (k) deals with health problems in their physical, psychological, social, cultural and existential dimensions.
2. *The specialty of general practice/family medicine.* General practitioners/family doctors are specialist physicians trained in the principles of the discipline. They are personal doctors primarily responsible for the provision of comprehensive and continuing care to every individual seeking medical care, irrespective of age, sex and illness. They care for individuals in the context of their family, their community and their culture, always respecting the autonomy of their patients. They recognise that they will also have a professional responsibility to their community. In negotiating management plans with their patients they integrate physical, psychological, social, cultural and existential factors, utilising the knowledge and trust engendered by

repeated contacts. General practitioners/family physicians exercise their professional role by promoting health, preventing disease, and providing cure, care or palliation. This is done either directly or through the services of others according to health needs and the resources available within the community that they serve, assisting patients where necessary in accessing these services. They must take responsibility for developing and maintaining their skills, personal balance and values as a basis for effective and safe patient care.

3. *The core competencies of the general practitioner/family doctor.* A definition of the discipline of general practice/family medicine and of the specialist family doctor must lead directly to the core competencies of the general practitioner/family doctor. 'Core' means essential to the discipline, irrespective of the healthcare system in which they are applied.

First, the 11 central characteristics that define the discipline relate to 11 abilities that every specialist family doctor should master. They can be clustered into six competencies (with reference to the characteristics listed above) as follows:

1. primary care management (a,b)
2. person-centred care (c,d,e)
3. specific problem-solving skills (f,g)
4. comprehensive approach (h,i)
5. community orientation (j)
6. holistic modelling (k).

Secondly, in order to practise the specialty, the competent practitioner implements these competencies in three areas:

1. clinical tasks
2. communication with patients
3. management of the practice.

Thirdly, as a person-centred scientific discipline, three background features should be considered as fundamental:

1. *contextual* – using the context of the person, the family, the community and their culture
2. *attitudinal* – based on the doctor's professional capabilities, values and ethics
3. *scientific* – adopting a critical and research-based approach to practice, and maintaining this through continuing learning and quality improvement.

The interrelationship between core competencies, implementation areas and fundamental features characterises the discipline and underlines the complexity of the specialty.

It is this complex interrelationship of core competencies that should guide and be reflected in the development of related agendas for teaching, research and quality improvement.

Chapter 3

'B' is for behaviour

The previous chapter defined the role of a family doctor as 'the set of values, norms and beliefs that she tries to adhere to – the principles that motivate her professional behaviour and actions'. As such, the role constitutes a set of drivers, some of which prompt behaviour that is appropriate to family doctors as a group, and the rest of which prompt the behaviour which enables each family doctor to do her job in her own personal way. The role that a family doctor chooses is thus of fundamental importance, but it is how the role is portrayed which actually does the work. As far as her patients are concerned, what is important is not what a family doctor intends to do, but what she does do.

This chapter discusses the behaviour – the 'B' of BARD – that might be used to portray the chosen role. For the purposes of this chapter, behaviour should be seen as the set of physical movements that a family doctor performs or the set of postures that she adopts while engaged in her professional work.

It is most unlikely that any single element of behaviour will ever express a family doctor's chosen role in its entirety. Different elements of behaviour are used to express different aspects of the role. In addition, it is unlikely for any given consultation that a family doctor will wish to portray her complete role, but rather she will portray only those aspects of the role that are appropriate to the occasion. In addition, a family doctor will often have a toolbox of different behaviours which portray the same aspect of her role – alternatives which can be employed either because the first-choice behaviour does not seem to be working, or because the family doctor wants to inject some variety into her consulting. Even when a role has been chosen, choices are still available right down the line – choices which are appropriate to individual consultations or strings of consultations. For example, what aspects of my role am I going to portray? What aspects of my role are appropriate to this patient at this time with this problem? What behaviour shall I use? What else can I try if the behaviour does not seem to be working?

The whole point of communication is what is received. Whatever your intention, if the information which is received does not accord with that intention, then the communication has failed. Some communications fail only partly, so that the transfer of information is incomplete. However, worse than this, sometimes efforts at communication can be misleading to the extent that entirely unintended information is transmitted. A family doctor needs to be a competent communicator, and it behoves her to make every effort to ensure that her communication is received 'loud and clear'. Techniques are available, drawn from sources as diverse as acting, neurolinguistics, human resource development and primary care medicine itself, to help people to communicate better. A family doctor must be familiar with and able to use these techniques if she is to offer effective consultations with her patients.

How to behave

The verb 'behave' has, according to the dictionary definition,[1] two related but distinct meanings:

'Conduct oneself, act'

and

'Conduct oneself with propriety.'

So 'behave' is what people do when they display behaviour, but the word also carries some moral overtones, as is evident in the phrase 'behave yourself' – it is how you *should* act. The way a person is expected to behave will depend on their age, sex, social status, education and any number of other factors. The point is that other people expect you to behave in a particular way – the appropriateness of behaviour is determined by society. Whether your behaviour accords with 'propriety' will depend on the circumstances. When you meet friends at a party, you do not behave towards them in the same way as you would towards the patients who attend your surgery. You do not behave towards your partner as you do towards your mother, or at least you don't if you want a quiet life.

Most behaviour has to be learned, and it continues to be learned throughout life. A limited number of pieces of non-verbal communication (NVC) are apparently inherent, but these are the exception.[2] If behaviour was not mainly learned, social behaviour could not be used as a measure of child development. Two-year-olds are expected to be selfish, demanding and thoughtless. Similar behaviour in a ten-year-old would raise questions about whether the child has a behavioural disorder, a problem which may sometimes be described as 'arrested development'.

Often an element of behaviour is used so much that it becomes second nature and is delivered without any apparent thought. It just 'feels right' to behave in a particular way in a particular situation. Elements of behaviour that have become internalised and intuitive are usually reliable because they will often have become intuitive for good reasons, through use and (presumably) successful use in the past. However, there will be consultation situations where for one reason or another intuitive behaviour does not work, and in such circumstances a family doctor must first be aware that the behaviour is not working, and secondly be sufficiently aware of what she is doing to enable the behaviour to be altered. Just because an element of behaviour is intuitive does not make it more 'natural' or 'honest'. An ability to adapt consulting behaviour to the requirements of the situation is the mark of an effective family doctor.

Put another way, if behaviour cannot be learned and altered by conscious effort, there is little point in trying to train anybody, let alone those on a family doctor specialist training scheme.

Communication consists mainly of actions rather than words. Linguistics – the words used – are responsible for only 7% of communication. Tonality or how the voice sounds is responsible for 38%, and physiology or body movements/posture account for the remaining 55%.[3] Nevertheless, a single element of behaviour will not be taken too seriously unless it is reinforced by other gestures or by what is said. NVC – or body language – is rather imprecise, and meaning is taken more from overall behaviour than from an individual mannerism or gesture.[2]

The eyes have it

There are at least two good reasons why a family doctor needs a working knowledge of NVC. Understanding NVC is a good way of working out what others are feeling and thinking, irrespective of what they might say, and so provides a kind of special insight into their thoughts. Hence NVC training is advocated for personnel work, management and sales. For a family doctor, a knowledge of NVC is a way of finding out what her patient is really thinking – a short cut to the 'hidden agenda'. An additional advantage of a family doctor understanding NVC is that, with training, different pieces of NVC can be emphasised or suppressed in order to improve communication with a patient. In fact, family doctors already use NVC (as indeed all people do) in all of their conversations. The challenge is to obtain an improvement in both perception and delivery.

Eye contact and direction of gaze are the most powerful sources of NVC.[2] Making eye contact with a patient (looking at their eyes and implicitly inviting them to look at your eyes) is particularly useful at the start of a consultation because it signals that you are seeking information, showing attention and interest, and inviting interaction. However, as the consultation proceeds, different rules apply. Keeping the contact too long – even a fraction of a second too long – suggests that you are seeking to control the consultation, or trying to dominate or threaten. These are consulting techniques that should only very rarely be used. Children who have not yet learned the rules of eye contact and do not know when to break off will sometimes be urged by a parent 'not to stare'. If eye contact is broken off too soon, this implies that you are being impolite, not paying attention, or being insincere, dishonest or shy.[2] If you break contact by looking downwards, this may be taken as indicating submission. Someone who is listening will look at the speaker between about one-third and two-thirds of the time. Making eye contact while talking implies that the speaker is seeking feedback to what has been said, or else it is a signal that an attitude is being revealed.

People who like each other tend to share greater eye contact. Conversely, sharing more eye contact makes people like each other more. This seems to be hard-wired into us, as quite tiny babies will respond positively to a steady gaze, and will even respond to fairly crudely drawn representations of eyes, such as a couple of small circles on a piece of paper. People who are of high social status, or who have charismatic 'star quality', tend to maintain more eye contact with the people to whom they are talking.[2]

The maintenance of eye contact and the direction of gaze are under conscious control, even if a continuous effort is needed to stop habitual patterns intruding. The size of the pupils is not under conscious control, but is a powerful indication that someone finds the object of their gaze attractive, and having dilated pupils tends to make people look more attractive. This was the reason for the use of deadly nightshade, *Atropa belladonna* (from the Italian, literally meaning 'fair lady') by women in the eighteenth century. And hence the phrase 'Dilated to meet you'.

Heads, we win

The two head movements worthy of particular attention are the nod and the head cock (a slight inclination to one side). When speaking, nods of the head can be used to punctuate what is being said, or (with other movements such as chin thrusts) to place emphasis on particular aspects of what is being said. When listening, single or double nods indicate that you are paying attention, and will tend to encourage the speaker to continue. Conversely, declining to nod is a disincentive and will probably result in the speaker cutting short their narrative. Synchronised nodding is a friendly gesture, a so-called *gestural echo*.

The head cock is an indication that you are listening attentively. This is another action that seems to be hard-wired, as small children and also dogs will cock their head when listening. Beginning a consultation with a posture that includes a cocked head will enable your patient to tell you more and talk for longer, if that is what you want.

A listener at the beginning of a spell of listening will quite quickly start to synchronise gestures with the speaker, and will then often assume a relaxed posture. As the speaker completes what they have to say (or when the listener wants to speak), the listener will continue their gestures but in a non-synchronous way, may interject some extra 'yes' and 'well' words, and may also signal their intent with a triple nod, not the single and double nods that are given by an encouraging listener. These are all useful forms of NVC for a family doctor who wants to move things along in a consultation.

In your face

A smile is an invitation to friendly interaction which appears to be understood in all cultures.[2] A smile is a broadening and uplifting of the mouth corners, possibly revealing the upper teeth, whereas a grimace which reveals the upper and lower teeth tends to look aggressive. Smiling has more impact on patients than it will have on fellow workers, and has more effect on women (who tend to be generally more sensitive to NVC) than on men. An additional advantage is that if you smile more, you will probably yourself feel in better spirits.

A smile is one of the 'big six' – the six basic facial expressions that have been discovered by research, namely happy, sad, disgusted, angry, afraid and inter-ested. Most people in most countries will interpret these expressions correctly. The happy smile has the most power and influence. People who use a greater range of facial expressions are regarded as more interesting and attractive.

On greeting another individual, a person will (as well as looking into the eyes) raise their eyebrows fleetingly. This *eyebrow flash* is pretty well understood all over the world as a greeting gesture.[2]

Deportment

An individual's repertoire of postures tends to be limited. Posture has a memory. For example, a person who has had significant problems with depression will tend to adopt a stooped and round-shouldered standing posture. Posture also reflects the current state of mind, so that someone who is feeling confident will stand up straight, with their chest out and their bottom in, but in a relaxed rather than military way. Facial expressions and posture intermix, so that the face reveals what the emotion is while the posture reveals the intensity of the emotion.

When sitting, leaning forward indicates that you are paying attention and are kindly disposed. Sitting back and to one side indicates benevolent relaxation, but sitting back straight can be perceived as a disgusted recoil. Attention to posture is also a good way of making the most of gestural echo – matching your posture to that of your patient is a good way of reinforcing rapport.

Steepling is a positioning of the hands as if in an attitude of prayer, with the fingertips together but the palms apart. This signifies confidence, or else a desire to make the listener think that you feel confident.

> John was never very keen on being video recorded when he was in training for family practice, but accepted that it had to be done. When he came to play back his first ever tape, the sound didn't work properly, so all he got was a visual picture of himself at work. He was appalled. He had imagined that he cut a dash as a young, relaxed, cheerful and sympathetic operator. What he saw was a slouched, balding figure approaching middle age, perched like a sack of potatoes in a soporific posture, wafting his overlong arms about in apparently meaningless activity.

Touch typing

A touch is a deliberate effort to make bodily contact. Some people like to be touched, and to touch, more than others. Men are more likely to initiate touch, but women are more likely to respond positively to a touch. Touching is more common during greetings and farewells.

Clearly the part of the body that is touched has to be chosen with care or else the touch will be misinterpreted. The acceptability of touch also depends on who is doing the touching – for instance, a mother's touch would be expected to be different from a friend's touch. Touch can be a very positive communication tool so long as the right person touches the right bit. A family doctor who feels that touching her patient will help a consultation (or who just feels like touching her patient) is safest if she restricts touching to the arms and shoulders.[2] The handshake, as well as being an example of touch, also has a role as an indication of good manners.

Legs

Leg positions do not contribute much to NVC, not because they are not important, but because interpretation of leg movements and positions is difficult. Many of the suggestions about the significance of various leg postures are of a quasi-sexual nature, since leg position determines the accessibility of genitalia and whether there is much thigh on view. In the consultation situation, a display of too much of the family doctor's crotch or thigh is to be avoided on the grounds of decency, but beyond this little can be read into leg positions. However, leg position is often observable as an example of gestural echo. During a consultation try crossing your legs and see how long it is before your patient crosses his legs as well.

Leakage is the phenomenon whereby unverbalised feelings are unwittingly revealed by body movements and positions. As with other forms of incontinence, the lower body is mainly involved. Tapping or twitching of the feet may indicate that something is being concealed, regardless of the words being used or the facial expressions being adopted.

Attractiveness and charisma

Those who are perceived by others to be attractive are also credited with other attributes. Attractive people are assumed to be talented, warm, responsive, kind, sensitive, interesting, poised, sociable and outgoing.[2] These are characteristics to which many family doctors would aspire in their professional and indeed personal lives. Warmer and more communicative relationships with patients are likely to result, so it would pay a family doctor to be as attractive to others as possible.

The 'rules' of being more attractive are fortunately entirely consistent with the 'rules' for encouraging patient involvement in a consultation.[2]

1. *Eye contact* – there should be as much as your patient appears comfortable with.
2. *Expressions* – let your face be lively and responsive, and smile a lot.
3. *Head movements* – single and double nods encourage your patient to speak. Most people like to talk about themselves, and encouraging them to do so will make them warm to you.
4. *Gestures* – use plenty (without actually waving your hands about), with no arm folding but plenty of open palm-up hand positions.
5. *Deportment* – this should be reasonably erect if you are standing, and if sitting use a forward-leaning symmetrical posture for listening and a backward-leaning asymmetrical posture for showing interest.
6. *Orientation (the angle at which family doctor and patient are interacting)* – see Chapter 5. Try to face your patient, and position yourself as close to them as possible without intruding.
7. *Touch* – use this as often as possible without causing offence.
8. *Appearance and physique* – dress like a family doctor. Being slim and having a soft-looking clear skin and clear eyes helps.
9. *Timing* – be sensitive to your patient's postures and movements, and mirror them. Try to move in time with your patient.
10. *Talking* – don't talk more than you listen, don't speak too fast or at the wrong volume, and try to avoid hesitations and other speech errors. Try to talk in complete sentences (*see* Chapter 6).

A family doctor who wants to appear impressive rather than just attractive would do well to watch how celebrities such as famous actors and 'pop stars' do it. Open gestures with the palms up and even outstretched arms abound. Touching is rare. The appearance is highly attractive and/or unusual. Timing is sharp, and they talk more than other people. By slight contrast, people of an aristocratic disposition use little in the way of gestures or facial expressions.

Frank was an independent city councillor as well as a local celebrity for his populist political work. Eventually his 20-a-day cigarette habit led to heart bypass surgery and then lung cancer, and he latched on to John as his family doctor for the last years of his life. John liked Frank, and was intrigued by his life as a local star. However, he never found consultations particularly comfortable, as Frank looked straight into his eyes all the time. This made John nervous, and he felt inferior. He also felt the need to fill any gaps in the conversation by talking, which made him repeat himself and lose his train of thought.

Manners

The most obvious examples of learned behaviours are displays of 'good manners' and courtesy. These are essentially meaningless elements of behaviour, or if they ever did have a meaning it has become lost in the depths of antiquity. We shake hands, even though it is some time since gentlemen stopped routinely carrying swords. We occasionally say 'How do you do?' to a patient, in the fervent hope that the enquiry will not produce a truthful reply.

Standing up when a patient enters or leaves the room, or when he offers a handshake, are small examples of courtesy which the family doctor should keep in mind for use. Helping patients on and off with their coats, or picking up their bags or walking sticks for them will, as well as displaying good manners, make the use of surgery time more efficient. A family doctor is probably on safest ground keeping the old courtesies alive – the young patients may think her stuffy and old-fashioned, but at least the elderly will not think her disgraceful.

Status

It might be assumed that communication is only effective between people who regard themselves as being of equal rank and status. However, this is not necessarily the case. Participants in a primary care consultation are never equal, but this does not mean that communication is always ineffective. The family doctor is the expert on primary care medicine, and the patient is the expert on what he believes and how he feels. In medical matters the family doctor has higher status, whereas in matters concerning the effects of the problem the patient has higher status. Each has their own equally important (but different) contribution to make to the consultation.

Looking at conversations generally, the people involved are almost never equal, and each individual has their own areas of expertise. In matters concerning their own knowledge, thoughts, feelings and opinions, they are of high status. Acting theory holds that all interactions between people contain at least an element of status projection.[4] Conversations as depicted on stage do not appear authentic if the participants look as though what they are saying lacks authority. People who believe that they are important may project high status all the time, but more generally a conversation rolls out as a *see-saw* where the participants are exhibiting a series of high-status and low-status elements of behaviour – one participant projects high-status behaviour while the other projects low-status behaviour, and then vice versa. The communication in a conversation is not impaired if the participants are of different status, so long as the relative status is accepted.[4]

Eric Berne, a medically trained writer, recognised the importance of status within doctor–patient interactions. The use within transactional analysis of the three 'ego states' of parent, adult and child is another formulation of the same thesis.[5] Being sensitive to the status relationships in a conversation is an effective way of improving communication. The projection of high status is not the same thing as taking control or manipulating. It can also be a way of preventing others from taking control of you. In addition, it is perfectly possible to take control of a situation or an interaction by projecting low status. For example, Berne describes a game called 'Little old me', most effectively played by old ladies:[5] 'I am old and sweet and rather pathetic, so don't ask me to do anything difficult or I will surely fail and let you down. I'll be nice to you and you must be nice to me.'

A person who is projecting high status will assume a relaxed posture, maintain eye contact and keep their head still when talking, and will speak in complete sentences and in a measured tone. This behaviour is entirely consistent with the behaviour exhibited by people who are considered to be attractive.[2] An assumption of low status is indicated by a stooped posture, averting the eyes, and speaking quickly and nervously with many verbal errors. This behaviour is often seen in people who are depressed and whose sense of self-worth is poor.

A family doctor must, when the circumstances require it, be prepared and able to project high status during a consultation. When important information has to be transmitted, a family doctor would do well to project high status while she is communicating this information. Patients in a consultation often do not behave as they would do in other interactions. Most patients apply their full attention and concentration during a consultation, excluding all other thoughts and activities. Many, for instance, seem to completely lose track of the passage of time. This mental state is similar to something that can occur during a theatrical performance, and which actors refer to as *trance*. During trance, people are very receptive to new ideas, but only from people whom they believe are of a higher status.[4] This is quite logical – why would a patient take advice from someone whom he believes does not know what she is talking about?

Trust

Consider some definitions of 'trust':

> a firm belief in the honesty, justice and strength of an individual or organisation.[6]

Or alternatively:

> an individual's belief that the sincerity, benevolence and truthfulness of another (or others) can be relied on.[7]

Or even:

> institutionalised optimism.[8]

Trust is an inevitable component of relationships between professionals of all kinds and the laity (i.e. the people who are outside the profession). A professional is someone who has undergone a course of higher training and has thereby acquired a useful skill that she will then use for the benefit of others, so a professional has knowledge and skills that not everyone possesses. The laity – those who have not undergone the training – therefore have to take it on trust that the professional will do her job properly and that her knowledge and skills are authentic.

Where trust exists, it can all too easily be disrupted when members of the profession – and often a very small number of members of the profession – act in an untrustworthy manner. The maintenance of trust is particularly important in the primary care setting, as the relationship that a family doctor and her patient achieve is an important factor in determining how likely the patient is to gain benefit from a consultation.[9]

> John was not looking forward to his next consultation with Alice, a small forthright woman in her seventies. John had been treating Alice for anaemia, but as all of her routine investigations were normal he had merely prescribed her some iron. However, John had just received a discharge summary from a seaside hospital. Alice had collapsed at her daughter's house and been admitted with a haemoglobin level of 6 g/dl. A silent peptic ulcer had been found, almost certainly caused by the non-steroidal agents that Alice had been taking for her osteoarthritis.
>
> John assumed that he was in for quite a roasting. After Alice had explained what happened, John grasped the nettle and apologised for what in retrospect was his prescribing error. He also said that he would understand if Alice decided to change family doctor. It was her reply that reinforced for John the value of years of consulting. She said 'No, I won't be doing that. I think too much of you.' The incident was never mentioned again.

The maintenance of trust is potentially more cost-effective than the alternatives.[7] Any legal contract or agreement which sought to cover all of the potential ramifications of a family doctor consultation would be at best simplistic or cumbersome, and at worst impossible to write. From the point of view of an economist:

> . . . all complex contracts are unavoidably incomplete, and they contain inevitable gaps, errors and omissions.[10]

Trust has both social and personal dimensions. Research suggests that the social components of trust (those which encourage the community of people to trust the community of family doctors) are based on the collective belief in the existence and value of the following:

- a just society (patients deserve to be treated fairly)
- moral integrity (family doctors do not do things only for their own interests)
- personal doctoring (family doctors focus their work on individual patients)

- sharing of power (patients are fellow human beings)
- compassion
- realistic medicine (don't promise what you cannot deliver)
- competence.[7]

Personal trust – that is, trust between a particular family doctor and a particular patient   is an extension of the social trust that society has in all family doctors. Consultation strategies have been identified which build up the personal trust that a patient has in a family doctor.[11]

- *Develop shared understanding and experience*. The use of general and personal conversation indicates that the family doctor is interested in the patient in terms of more than just medical matters.
- *Demonstrate willingness to co-operate*. The family doctor volunteers and freely shares information, and so engages in a reciprocal relationship.
- *Competence development*. Emphasising the competence of the patient and under-playing the family doctor's own contribution puts the consultation interaction on a more equal footing.

A study from UK family practice found that 76% of patients reported high levels of trust in their family doctor. Trust was strongly related to the quality of the family doctor–patient relationship, specifically communication, interpersonal care and knowledge of the patient. In this study, duration of registration with the family doctor and the proportion of visits to the usual family doctor were not correlated with levels of trust.[12] Family doctors appear to earn the trust of their patients through the quality of their communication rather than through just getting older together. Patients are accepting that continuity of care in the old sense – that is, an individual family doctor being available at all times – is no longer part of primary care medicine.

The trust that patients have in their family doctor is contingent not only on the knowledge that the doctor has, but also on how she uses it. The knowledge that a family doctor has is no longer exclusive, and is readily accessible to the public at large, so that a patient will now often know more about their disease and its treatment than does their family doctor. However, the way in which a family doctor uses her knowledge remains different and special. By their continuing level of trust, family practice patients clearly recognise the importance of the thinking and problem-solving skills of the generalist, even if medical information can be obtained elsewhere.

Trust is of course a two-way process. Family doctors trust their patients to tell the truth about their symptoms, to let them know if illness is likely, not to waste time, and to take some responsibility for and co-operate with treatment. In a family doctor consultation the patient has knowledge that the family doctor wants, and the family doctor has knowledge that the patient wants, so the trust is mutual.

Respecting and maintaining the trust of their patients remains an important responsibility for family doctors. It is the traditions of family practice – family doctors who do the things that family doctors have always done – which reinforce the trust that patients have in their family doctor.

> Only in the archaeology of general practice can we find our basic values and the capacity to carry us into the future.[7]

John really had no time for Eric, a regular attender with a body full of aches and pains that were clearly primarily of psychological origin. Eric always declined psychological help, while insisting on numerous X-rays and 'strong' pain-killing medications. He had not worked for years despite appearing to be in rude good health, and always blamed others for his plight. It was difficult to feel empathy with him.

At the end of a particularly trying consultation, John tried confrontation (never his strongest suit). He told Eric that it must be obvious that they were getting nowhere, that they completely disagreed about the right way forward, and that he had no sympathy for Eric's intransigent attitudes. He closed by asking *'So why do you keep coming to see me?'* *'Because you're my doctor, aren't you?'* Eric replied.

Expressing emotion

Even when armed with a thorough knowledge of NVC, a family doctor will on occasion want to express an emotion with particular effect during a consultation. Sympathy may be needed when consulting with a bereaved patient. Concern may be needed when you want to reassure a somatising patient that you are taking his physical symptoms seriously. Just occasionally anger may be needed if you feel that a patient has behaved in an unacceptable way. Most interactions between people have an emotional content, and the freedom and confidence to express emotions is a valuable consultation tool if a conversation between a family doctor and her patient is to be a relaxed and fruitful event.

The forceful expression of emotion is not something that comes particularly easily to family doctors, especially those who spend most of their professional life trying to be calm and collected. The behaviour that is used must appear authentic or it will not properly express the desired emotion. Learning and presenting new emotional behaviour in an effective and realistic way is something that actors do all the time.

A family doctor who is searching for a suitable behaviour to express an emotion might find it helpful to consider Stanislavsky's advice to aspiring actors in his concept of *emotion memory*.[13] An actor who is trying to portray a particular emotion or feeling in an authentic way needs a form of behaviour that will convince the audience, that is consistent with the role being enacted, and that is also consistent with the inherent personality of the actor. The actor who is preparing to portray an emotion is encouraged to reflect on a time when they experienced the required feeling or emotion in their own life, and to recall in as much detail as possible what words and actions they used. Such behaviour will be a natural expression of that emotion for that particular actor, and this contributes to the effectiveness of the portrayal. A refinement is for the actor to try to relive the emotion during the actual performance, so that it may be portrayed more convincingly. 'Acting' classes as such do not figure in the curriculum of most drama schools.[14] What actors in training are taught is the tools with which to access the experiences that they have already had, and the elements of behaviour that they have already exhibited. Learning to act is a process of finding out about oneself.

A family doctor can also use emotion memory to create fresh elements of behaviour for her professional use. When an emotion has been chosen which is consistent with the words that are to be used in a consultation, the family doctor then goes back in her own experience to a time when she spontaneously felt that emotion for real. Recalling the NVC used, this can be replicated for the consultation. The NVC which is being used is real for that family doctor, so the portrayal will be realistic and convincing. When the recalled NVC has been used a few times, it too will become internalised and more readily available for use in future consultations.

> John was finding dealing with one of the partners in his family practice increasingly wearisome, an opinion that was shared by the remaining partners. At meetings, the errant partner would talk endlessly, often into the small hours of the morning, until everyone else gave up and let him have his own way. John felt that poor decisions were being made that only one of the partners really agreed with.
>
> During a typical exchange, John felt some genuine anger rising within him, but instead of suppressing it (as was his habit as a sober professional), he decided quite consciously to give the emotion its head to see what would result. After a brief but loud tirade, the offending partner backed down completely. His partners told John afterwards that during his brief excursion into the emotional unknown John was wide-eyed and sweating, and looked and sounded the true incarnation of anger. He was slightly embarrassed.

Some readers will find the idea of deliberately using elements of behaviour to further a consultation potentially dishonest and unethical. This topic will be returned to in Chapter 8.

Applied behaviour

How does all of this information fit in with a normal consultation in primary care? Consider, for example, a fairly typical consultation for vertigo in a patient who is not only distressed by his symptoms, but also concerned that this might be the beginning of a stroke. The consulting family doctor's chosen role includes wanting to be attractive to and inspire confidence in her patients, but also includes wanting to be understanding and reassuring. In addition, she is mindful of the over-arching principle of her role that she should be clinically proficient.

- The family doctor will stand erect and greet her patient from the waiting room with a smile and a lift of the eyebrows. A well-known patient may also get a handshake or a pat on the shoulder.
- When both are seated the doctor may (with a familiar patient) continue the smile and eye contact, while leaning back and to the side and exchanging a few seconds of pleasantries about the weather.
- As business starts she will turn to face her patient, lean forward with her head

slightly cocked, her hands folded in her lap and her knees nearly together, and use an opening verbal gambit such as 'What can I do for you today?'.

- While listening to the narrative she will maintain eye contact, but not all the time so as not to embarrass her patient, and she will keep the consultation going with nods of her head in time with the flow of words. Even though the problem does not sound too bad, she may use a facial expression of empathy which she first found herself using when her son's pet rabbit had died, and which she has used subsequently in other consultations to good effect. She may shift her posture to echo that of her patient.
- When she has heard enough and/or her patient seems to have finished what he wanted to say, the family doctor might break eye contact, nod her head three times, and add some extra verbal interjections to signal that she now wants her say. During the questions phase she may continue to lean forward or else she may try the asymmetrical backward-leaning posture.
- As the family doctor has already read the chapter on room (*see* Chapter 5) in this book, she may stand at this point to signal that an examination is to take place. She will use suitable equipment and instruments to secure the diagnosis and to allay her patient's concerns about having a stroke.
- Settling back in her seat, she will regain eye contact and steeple her fingers while explaining her findings and discussing the probable diagnosis. She will inspire the confidence of her patient by sitting still and keeping her head still, and by talking in complete sentences and measured tones.
- Management options may be offered, after which the doctor will support her chin with the thumb and first two fingers of one hand until a response to her suggestions is forthcoming and a management plan agreed.
- The doctor will sign the prescription with a flourish, fold it and hand it to the patient.
- She will then stand and, while helping her patient on with his coat, go through the agreed management plan once more. She will hold the door open and the parting may possibly be accompanied by a further handshake or a pat on the shoulder.

Summary

The majority of communication is achieved through behaviour rather than words. Behaviour is the means by which intentions are manifested to the outside world. The behaviour that is used will depend on the family doctor's chosen role, and individual elements of behaviour can be learned either socially (such as manners and deportment), by trial and error, or by deliberately recalling personal life experiences ('emotion memory'). Family doctors still enjoy high status, at least in the context of their work, and that status must be accepted and utilised rather than wished away. Trust remains an important component of the complex interaction that consulting in family practice represents, and the wise doctor will take steps to respect, maintain and deserve that trust.

References

1. Fowler HW and Fowler FG (eds) (1974) *The Concise Oxford Dictionary.* Oxford University Press, Oxford.
2. Wainwright GR (2003) *Teach Yourself Body Language.* Hodder & Stoughton, London.
3. Walter J and Bayat A (2003) Neurolinguistic programming: verbal communication. *BMJ Careers.* **15 March:** s83.
4. Johnstone K (1981) *Impro.* Methuen, London.
5. Berne E (1964) *Games People Play.* Penguin, Harmondsworth.
6. Maynard A and Bloor K (2003) Trust, performance management and the new GP contract. *Br J Gen Pract.* **53**: 754–5.
7. Fugelli P (2001) Trust – in general practice. *Br J Gen Pract.* **51**: 575–9.
8. Browning G (2003) How to . . . trust. *Guardian.* **23 August:** 10.
9. Silverman J, Kurtz S and Draper J (2004) *Skills for Communicating with Patients* (2e). Radcliffe Publishing, Oxford.
10. Williamson OE (2002) The theory of the firm as governance structure: from choice to contract. *J Econ Perspect.* **16**: 171–95.
11. Alaszewski A and Horlick-Jones T (2003) How can doctors communicate information about risk more effectively? *BMJ.* **327**: 728–31.
12. Tarrant C, Stokes T and Baker R (2003) Factors associated with patients' trust in their general practitioner: a cross-sectional survey. *Br J Gen Pract.* **53**: 798–800.
13. Morrison H (1998) *Acting Skills.* A&C Black, London.
14. Jones E (1998) *Teach Yourself Acting.* Hodder Headline, London.

Chapter 4

'A' is for aims

A sense of direction

The ongoing healthcare relationship between a family doctor and her patient – whether a single consultation, a series of consultations or a lifetime – must have a direction or some idea of where it is going. Indeed the relationship will be characterised not by a single direction but by a multitude of directions, pathways along which the journey will result in one or more desired outcomes. It may for instance be desirable for a patient to lose weight, take more exercise, have a lower blood pressure and smoke fewer cigarettes – linked but independently valuable directions of change. Some directions are valid in the short term, some in the medium term and some in the long term. Directions may lose priority with time, and just as assuredly others will emerge, especially over a long-term relationship.

There have to be directions of travel because, with the exception of attendances for routine disease surveillance, patients tend to consult a family doctor when they want to change something about themselves. Their present position is characterised by symptoms and concerns. Where a patient wants to be is in a position without symptoms and concerns. He wants to move from his present position to a better one.

The direction or directions of a healthcare relationship should be as explicit as possible. A family doctor and her patient will have different agendas for their consultation, agendas that reflect the specific needs and aspirations of each of them. These agendas will to a large degree overlap, but they will nonetheless be different. Such differences can prove very disruptive. If the direction of a consultation is transparent, it can be offered for discussion and amendment. Being open and specific about the intended direction of the consultation means that the family doctor can agree the direction with her patient. It is best if the family doctor and the patient are both singing from the same hymn-sheet.

> Dennis, a timid man in his seventies, had been seeing John because of nocturia. His prostate felt large but not malignant, but his prostate-specific antigen was elevated to a level where the local protocol suggested that a referral was in order. At the outpatient clinic he was offered a prostate biopsy, but declined even though he was scared of having cancer. Dennis's wife had had a stroke, and was utterly dependent on Dennis for her care. She could go into a nursing home while Dennis had his surgery and recovered, but Dennis knew that she would not like this. When Dennis's true feelings emerged, John agreed to check his PSA at regular intervals, on the understanding that if the level rose further the biopsy would become urgent.

Stakeholders in the consultation

This chapter is about aims – the 'A' of BARD. For the purposes of this chapter, 'aims' are the directions along which a family doctor wants to progress a consultation or a series of consultations.

When setting aims for a consultation it is necessary to decide who has a legitimate interest in the consultation. On whose behalf are the aims being set? Each consultation in family practice has implications for more people than just the immediate participants, and each of these stakeholders has a right to be considered when aims are being decided.

- The patient is the person who has first call on what happens in a consultation, and is quite properly the main focus of attention. The training that family doctors and others undergo, and the organisation and infrastructure that are set up, all have patient care as a primary aim. Consultations should be 'patient centred'.[1] The patient comes first.
- The family doctor has a legitimate vested interest in what happens during a consultation. A family doctor in a consultation has an obligation to translate patient wants into patient needs. Setting an aim or aims for a consultation is something for which the family doctor takes primary responsibility. It is the family doctor who is likely to have a wider appreciation of which aims are likely to be relevant and appropriate. It is also the family doctor who is more aware of the options, and who is trusted through her professional position to make a decent job of pursuing the agreed option. In addition, family doctors spend much more of their time consulting than do individual patients – to a family doctor consulting is a very important part of life.
- The company of family doctors – the profession as a whole – has an interest in how each individual family doctor behaves and does her work. Family doctors should behave as family doctors are supposed to behave. Keen public interest in the tiny minority who fall foul of the medical disciplinary procedures emphasises the fact that, to the public, one bad family doctor reflects badly on all family doctors. The reliability of the regulatory framework within which family doctors work is essential not only to ensure patient trust, but also to justify the professional status of all family doctors. Family doctors who do not behave like family doctors run the risk of causing disruption to their patients and peers.
- Only a minority of healthcare workers are family doctors. However, other staff have an interest in what goes on, because they are affected by the results. Decisions to refer or investigate have clear implications for the people accepting the referrals or processing the investigations. In primary care, the reception staff (and nowadays often the nurses) rather than the family doctors are really on the front line, and absorb much of the pressure on the service. Managers are needed to keep the whole show on the road, and health is equally their profession and career.
- The delivery of healthcare has organisational needs. The processes used to deliver care are integral to the overall quality of that care. Individual family doctor or patient preference may occasionally be less important than the need for the organisation to operate smoothly for all concerned.
- The rest of the patients who are looked after by the family practice deserve

consideration. A prolonged consultation may be welcomed by the patient involved, but can also stretch the charitable feelings of those in the waiting room to an unacceptable degree. In a situation of limited resources, one patient using a service may lead to another who cannot, or who has to wait longer in order to use it.

- Society at large also has an interest. The people who make up society know that they will be patients themselves some day – everyone is a potential consumer. In many countries the taxpayer is a stakeholder since at least a proportion, if not nearly all, of healthcare expenditure is supported through taxation. The politicians who aspire to speak for and act on behalf of their electorate must juggle the needs of healthcare with the other services for which they are responsible.

A patient in a consultation is the main originator of patient-centred aims, and will also usually have some opinions about the rights of other stakeholders. Patients are not oblivious to the interests of other patients or the smooth running of the healthcare organisation. However, a family doctor in consultation may well have a rather broader understanding of the potential competing interests, and is custodian of the rights of the wider range of stakeholders. Just how much account she takes of other stakeholders will be determined by her own particular set of principles – for instance, what one family doctor will regard as 'legitimate interest', another will view as 'meddlesome interference'.

Aims and targets

The setting of aims for a consultation is the method by which a family doctor can apply to individual patient contacts both her own professional role and her understanding of the interests of all the stakeholders to the consultation. However, it is the two immediate participants in a consultation – the family doctor and the patient – who finally agree which aims to pursue. When a family doctor and her patient are in accord about which way to go, the consultation can then be genuinely collaborative.

An 'aim' defines direction in much the same way as choosing a compass bearing when travelling. Features on the health landscape that are passed along the way may be noteworthy, but they do not distract from the overall purpose of the journey. On the other hand, setting a 'target' or a series of targets is like choosing the points through which the journey should pass. It is assumed that the purpose of the journey will be achieved by reaching each target.

Aims are more useful than targets. The use of 'targets' in the primary healthcare setting is unbiological, unscientific, jeopardises the mental health of care workers, offers perverse incentives and encourages shoddy management. Is this an overly harsh view? Perhaps a few words of justification are in order.

- An 'aim' defines the direction of progress with rather more precision than a 'target'. Consider, for instance, the management of a patient with diabetes. The aim is to move glycaemic control towards normal. A possible target may be to secure normal blood sugar readings at the diabetic clinic. Some patients will be tempted during the two weeks before a clinic visit to keep to their diet and be sure to take the medication properly so that the reading on the day is declared normal. This of course rather misses the point. The target has become more important than the aim. Having a target encourages people to devise ways to get round it by whatever circuitous route they can find, but an aim will not permit such pointless invention.

- A target is a threshold imposed on what may be in biological terms a situation of continuous variation. Smoking 19 rather than 20 cigarettes a day is a worthwhile change. A little exercise may not be as beneficial as a lot of exercise, but it is still better than no exercise at all. Research has been unable to define the 'right' blood sugar level or blood pressure for a diabetic, for it seems that lower is better. The idea of having aims rather than targets reflects biological reality. An attempt to impose artificial targets invites the criticism that the targets are being promoted for reasons other than patient well-being.
- The scientific evidence often does not support the imposition of targets. For a target to be justified at all, it must be supported by reliable evidence. As well as the previous reservation about imposing targets on continuous variation, there is the additional problem that much of the available evidence relates to populations rather than to individuals, and family doctors work with individuals. Why is the official safe alcohol limit for an eight-stone man the same as that for a 20-stone man? Why do only a minority of heavy users of alcohol end up with liver damage? Why do half of cigarette smokers not die of their habit? Which is the half that will die?
- Targets may generate perverse incentives. Once a target has been met, there is less reason to exceed it, and an evidently unattainable target is not worth pursuing at all. A target may be set merely because it is possible to set it, and not because achievement of the target is more important than another health objective that doesn't happen to be the subject of a target.
- Targets can promote either complacency or a sense of failure. Complacency may result when a target has been achieved, whatever the legitimacy of the target. The existence of the target sets its own agenda. On the other hand, not reaching the target can result in despondency. Given the current mental health vulnerability of family doctors, this cannot be good news.
- On the wider stage of healthcare organisation, target setting encourages a low grade of management from whoever it is that sets the target. Once set, a target can be simply tightened year on year. This does little to address the real problems of patients and their family doctors, who need a more thoughtful and competent management input.

The people who promote the use of targets in healthcare argue that target setting has a proven track record in many management settings of achieving – well – the targets. It is not just within healthcare that the limitations of targets are recognised, and it is apparent that the factors which impair the effectiveness of target setting in healthcare are just the same as those which impair it in other disciplines.[2]

Targets are more memorable than aims, and for this reason are sometimes used by family doctors in clinical situations. If advice is offered to a patient, the more specific and concrete that advice is, the more likely it is to be remembered and adhered to. By all means set targets for the short term, but do not be deluded into thinking that they are any more than stepping-stones in pursuit of longer-term aims.

Quality of service

When agreeing aims with a patient during a consultation, the family doctor must bear in mind that most patients are not in a position to accurately evaluate the technical quality of the service that they are receiving. They know something about outcomes because it is they who have the symptoms, but looking only at patient symptoms is an incomplete way of evaluating the quality of the process of healthcare delivery. It is quite possible for a family doctor to do everything right, and yet for her patient to feel no better – 'the operation was a success, but the patient died'. Perversely, it is also possible to do everything wrong and still be showered with praise by your patient. Some patients get better because of treatment from their family doctor, and some patients get better in spite of it. A patient may want – nay expect – a high-quality service, but there may not be agreement between the family doctor and the patient about what constitutes a high-quality service.

This is not to say that patients have no perception of quality, just that they are probably using criteria which are different, and of which the family doctor may be completely unaware. Patients tend to use proxy measures of quality of service – the things that they can appreciate.[3] Examples include the following.

- Are appointments kept on time?
- Does the diagnosis prove to be accurate?
- Is there a minimum of waiting?
- Is there a willingness to listen?
- How many letters have the practitioners got after their names?
- Is the building appropriate for the task?
- Do the staff look efficient and behave efficiently?
- Was the family doctor nice to me?
- Was I acknowledged as a person?
- Did I feel rushed?

A family doctor who does not have due regard for these factors runs the risk of having an unhappy patient, however technically competent the medical service delivered may have been.

Other providers of highly technical services also face this problem of clients who do not appreciate the quality of the service that they are receiving. Research on lawyers suggests that only 15% of how happy or unhappy a client is with their performance can be predicted from the outcome of the case, but 60% of the variance can be attributed to how courteous or discourteous the client perceives the lawyer to have been. Qualities such as reliability, responsiveness, assurance (knowledge, courtesy and the ability to inspire trust) and empathy all contribute to the customer's perception of the quality of the service.[3]

If there is agreement between the family doctor and the patient about the aim that is being pursued – if the aims of the consultation are shared – then a satisfied patient is more likely to result. This requires the family doctor and the patient to openly discuss their perspectives on what should be done. It is the family doctor who will normally be in a better position to judge what is possible rather than what would be desirable.

The other factors that contribute to perceived quality are *tangibles* – the physical facilities, equipment, personnel and written materials that the customer encounters.[3] This subject is discussed further in Chapter 5.

> John was devastated when he received his first complaint. He had been asked to visit a patient with a chest infection urgently on a Sunday afternoon. He had attended within 30 minutes of the call, dispensed some antibiotics from his bag, and telephoned three days later to learn that his patient was much better. The substance of the complaint was that John had been 'improperly dressed' for the visit because he was not wearing a tie.

Categories of aims

The delivery of technically competent medical care is only a small part of what happens in a consultation – legitimate aims for a consultation are of much broader scope than the simply biomedical. There are many stakeholders. It is alright for a family doctor to want things from her consultations. It is alright to keep in mind the organisational integrity of the practice. It is alright to watch out for what the politicians, managers and lawyers are doing.

Patient aims

The priority for a family doctor in consultation is to find out what her patient wants and what his aims are. Sometimes a patient will want something that is not possible, in which case it is the family doctor's job to explain the practicalities. A consultation will nearly always end up generating options for different but acceptable (or tolerable) management plans. A family doctor may consider one option to be the best, and may therefore be reluctant to countenance alternatives. However, in all but the most dangerous circumstances it is for the patient to make his choice, armed with all of the relevant information about the benefits and drawbacks of each option. This is the essence of *informed consent*.

> Whenever John got the chance, he liked to chat with the community mental health nurses about his ongoing cases. During one discussion he was moaning about a woman he had been seeing who was attending at ever more frequent intervals without an obvious reason, and John expressed a fear that she was becoming dependent on him. The nurse's reply surprised him. *'Why does it worry you that she is becoming dependent?'*, she asked. *'I know this woman, and she has spent her life looking for someone to depend on. At least you are more reliable than some of the people she has chosen in the past.'*

Clinical aims

The *therapeutic aims* of a consultation include history taking, examination, investigation, prescribing and referral. Further clinical aims might be termed *communication aims*, namely the effective use of behavioural and communication skills intended to result in optimum clinical management. In short, the overall clinical aim is to get the diagnosis and treatment plan right. This area is extremely well covered in detail by existing 'task-based' models of the family doctor consultation.

Professional aims

Maintaining the integrity of the relationship that patients in general have with family doctors in general is a legitimate aim of all consultations. This relationship provides an essential framework for the way in which family doctors and patients generally interact – the behavioural ground rules for a consultation. Each family doctor will wish to express her professionalism in her own unique way, but it is not possible to enter a consultation with a patient who has no preconceptions about how the doctor is expected to behave. Some of this framework can be regarded as *anthropological* – the mutual understanding that relationships between healers and patients have developed over thousands of years of history and tradition.

A family doctor who behaves – and moreover is seen to behave – in an ethical manner promotes her professional image. A family doctor should be trustworthy, competent and honest. In other words, a family doctor should make every effort to behave in a way that does not attract the interest of the police, the lawyers or the professional regulatory body. Such *medico-legal aims* might include the equally pressing aim not to get prosecuted, sued or struck off.

Social aims

It is reasonable for a family doctor who is involved in patient consultations for maybe five or six hours a day not to want those consultations to be characterised by negative emotions such as anger, conflict and frustration. Maintaining cordial relations with patients is a legitimate aim. For their part, patients usually welcome a little social content to their consultations,[4] and similarly do not wish their consultation experience to be unnecessarily unpleasant. A family doctor and her regular patients will have had time to build their relationship beyond the simply biomedical.[4.1]

[4.1] In the days when the spiritual was dominant over the scientific, illness was widely regarded as the result of supernatural forces. If the deity or deities were so disposed, they would confer pain and misery on their subjects. If such a belief is held, it is logical that the roles of priest and healer should overlap, since appeasing the deity is a good way of getting rid of symptoms. In some traditions the healer was only concerned with relieving illness, not with trying to avoid death. Death, the transition from life to something else, was felt to be a wholly spiritual issue which mankind should not deign to interfere with.[5] Is it stretching credulity to think that the remnants of such beliefs are still at work? If the technicalities of what a family doctor does are beyond the understanding of the majority of her patients, then her patient has to believe both in the validity of the skills that the doctor possesses, and also that she will use those skills beneficently. In such a context, good health is part of the family doctor's gift, something that she chooses to bestow or withhold, so it is sensible for patients to try to keep their family doctor friendly. Conversely, a patient who believes that he is on cordial terms with his family doctor is also likely to believe that he is getting a good-quality service from her. It is sensible for the family doctor to promote an atmosphere of friendliness when consulting.

In his own training family practice, John had got used to the fact that his trainer was something of a local celebrity. One of his abiding memories was of being taken by his trainer to the Annual General Meeting of the local chrysanthemum society of which his trainer was president that year. John's trainer knew nothing about and had no interest in chrysanthemums, but was asked to be president as he was the nearest thing the local community had to a dignitary.

The social nature of the relationship can be promoted by a family doctor who remembers her patient's significant social events, such as births, deaths, and family illnesses and misfortunes. Further benefit may be obtained by a family doctor who is forthcoming about her own family, holidays, interests, etc. Some family doctors will feel more comfortable talking to their patients in this way than others. However, for those who feel able to make such gestures of closeness to their patients, the rewards in terms of improved relationships can be considerable. In addition, it is surprising how much interesting stuff patients know.

Organisational aims

The following epigram is famously attributed to Joseph Stalin: 'Once the political line has been settled, organisation counts for all.' Knowing what to do is only half the battle – it is also important to get it done. The healthcare systems in all of the economically advanced countries are large organisations. For example, the UK National Health Service is by some margin the biggest employer in the country. Larger family practices may look after tens of thousands of patients, and turn over considerable sums of money. All of this has to be managed and organised. Consultation aims that cover such issues as processes, staff relationships and the use of time and money are all legitimate considerations in individual consultations.

John had always regarded patient groups as self-evidently a good thing. Patients have a right to more say in how their medical services are organised, and could well have many good ideas about how to do things better. So John invited to a meeting a group of patients who had been nominated by the other doctors in his family practice. These patients were all 'regulars' at the surgery, and each of them had their own agenda relating to their own illness. Indeed many had been nominated by the other doctors as a way of taking the heat off themselves.

Over the course of four meetings, each patient took the opportunity to describe their own problems in some detail. The only ideas that were forthcoming were to do with better access to new treatments, and all of the participants were too disabled to do any useful work for the group. Eventually John let the group lapse – with a heavy heart about his first real foray into patient autonomy, and having learned a few home truths about the internal politics of how a family practice works.

Personal aims

As if that were not enough, each family doctor will have one or more personal aims for each consultation. Some of these aims will relate to relations with that patient.

- Do I want this patient to feel relaxed and comfortable, or to be aware of the time they are taking?
- Am I after a 'stroke' (in transactional analysis terms) from this patient, so that he will tell me what a good family doctor I am?
- Do I actually like being in this patient's company, or do I wish that he would go and see somebody else?

Other personal aims are to do with the specific reputation that the family doctor wants to have among patients generally.

- Do I want to appear friendly, or businesslike and efficient?
- Should I look calm, or should I allow myself to appear harassed and stressed?
- Which of my principles am I trying to display prominently?

Further aims are concerned with survival. These aims are part of what Neighbour calls 'housekeeping'.[6]

- Am I ready to face the next patient?
- Can I get through the surgery in time so that I can pick up the children from school?
- Can I get through the surgery unscathed, or even only mildly scathed?
- Should I try and see the next patient before having that cup of coffee, or going to the toilet?
- Can I retire yet?

> David was a superannuated hippy. After his sociology degree and a failed marriage, he had become a railway signalman until the disability of his ankylosing spondylitis caught up with him. He now spent his time gardening and going on ecological field trips. He developed some breathlessness and a low-grade depression after his mother died, and had several consultations with John over a period of two years, during which no progress appeared to be made. David was witty, erudite and deeply moral – qualities that John admired. To get over his professional frustration at the lack of progress, John decided that during David's visits to the surgery he would pretend they were meeting at a pub.

A 'good enough' consultation

Clearly, the number of aims that it might be possible to pursue in each consultation is enormous. So which do you choose? And how do you know when to stop? How good is 'good enough'? What standard of consultation will leave a family doctor secure in the belief that she has done right by her patients, and is up to speed with her colleagues? When is it reasonable either to defer until the future or to defer permanently?

A book by the gloriously named Bruno Bettelheim – he is, as you might expect, an American child psychologist – gave me much solace when our daughters were young. *A Good Enough Parent*[7] points out that all parents feel guilty about the standard of their parenting efforts, and all fear that their children will turn out delinquent as a result. The book also points out that in most cases the parents are wrong, and their children turn out just fine (or at least as 'fine' as previous generations). Despite their fears, most parents are doing their job sufficiently well to secure a reasonable result.

Most family doctors will have similar fears that they are not doing their job properly, and that their patients are suffering as a result. In an individual consultation, most of the possible tasks are always left undone. Possibly working in isolation, each family doctor is not sure that her performance is up to standard – this is one reason why appraisal and peer discussion can be such useful and reassuring educational tools. Yet the reality is that most family doctors are doing a perfectly good job most of the time. They all make the occasional mistake, but very few family doctors are so consistently under-performing that their fitness to practise is called into question. People are living longer, and are staying healthy longer. Whatever family doctors are doing it must be a step in the right direction. You could always have done a consultation better, but you could also have done it a lot worse.

So how many aims is it reasonable to try and fulfil during a consultation? If there are too few aims, patients are not getting a fair share. Having too many aims risks failure of one or more of them, with attendant disappointment, frustration and guilt. And there is a limit – even for women – to how many problems can be 'multi-tasked' at any one time. The difficulty of an act of juggling depends on the number of balls in use.

An overriding priority for every consultation must be patient safety, whatever else may go on. Thus a family doctor must be sure that she can recognise and deal with a heart attack or a perforated duodenal ulcer. It also means that she should find out about suicide risk.

Beyond securing patient safety, I would suggest that in every consultation a family doctor should try to pursue a maximum of four aims, at least one of which should be clinical. In some consultations it is not possible to pursue more than a single aim, but in most cases there is scope for one or two more. And once safety has been secured and a maximum of four aims have been pursued, then stop.

Which of the many possible aims should be pursued? The aims that are pursued should be the ones that the family doctor and the patient agree are most important. Many patients will of course (and it feels as if they are doing this in increasing numbers) present more than one problem at a consultation. The average patient will enter a consultation with between one and four concerns.[3] As long as all of the concerns are revealed at an early stage in the consultation, it should be possible to amalgamate those that are in fact the same problem, and for the family doctor and her patient to prioritise the list of consultation aims accordingly. Such prioritisation will need to take account of her patient's priorities as well as her own. Access to primary care teams remains staggeringly good (just try and get an appointment with your bank manager or hairdresser within 48 hours), which means that deferred problems are not deferred for too long.

The question to ask with regard to whether a consultation is complete is not then 'What is best?', but 'What is reasonable?'. The abolition of all symptoms and death is not an option. Family doctors facilitate a process – they do not achieve a particularly definable goal. Family doctors keep people going. Of course the family doctor owes it to herself, her profession and her patients to do the best job she can, but that does not include aiming so high that every consultation brings renewed disappointments.

- Some aims are impossible to achieve. It is not unusual to have 'wishes' for patients, such as 'I wish this lady did not have cancer'. Such wishes are impossible to deliver, and should not be called 'aims'.
- Some aims cannot be achieved because they require too much time and other resources. It is not unusual for a family doctor to feel that she would like more time with each patient, and more energy to invest in their care. Much musculoskeletal pain could probably be relieved by prompt physical therapy, but this is not going to happen if the practice physiotherapist is off work with a bad back and already has a six-month routine waiting list.
- Some aims cannot be achieved because of patient and/or family doctor attitudes. For example, keen athletes often do not take kindly to suggestions that rest might be an appropriate treatment for their latest injury. A family doctor who believes that addictive behaviour is a moral problem rather than a medical one is unlikely to want to provide treatment for heroin abuse.

> John found that he was regularly irritated by parents who failed to control their patently healthy offspring in the surgery, who could not get them to sit still and be quiet while they were examined, or who moaned about petty sleeping problems. It said in the books that parenting was hard work, but surely a little more fortitude, moral backbone and consistent discipline would bring the little darlings into line. His motivations told him to be caring and understanding, but he frequently found himself thinking in terms of 'over-anxious parents'. Then John had children of his own.

- Sometimes an aim cannot be achieved because the time is not right. It is neither appropriate nor realistic to put pressure on a recently bereaved widow to stop smoking.

> John had become quite attached to June, a teacher who had had to retire early because she was unable to stop overworking, and who was now constantly stressed by caring for her elderly sister. Because of a previous alcohol problem, she had ended up on significant doses of psychotropic medication, including benzodiazepines.
>
> John's agreement with June was that the benzodiazepines should be gradually withdrawn, but at each monthly meeting there was always a reason not to do so – for example, June had been tempted to restart her

Continued

heavy drinking or her sister was ill. John realised that one of the reasons why there was no progress was that his enjoyment of his chats with June and his desire to stay on friendly terms with her had become as important as what he knew to be medically desirable. Once he had shared this observation with June, their consultations became much more productive, as June seemed convinced that what John suggested to her was actually in her best interests.

Is this practicable?

Adding all of these potential aims to the established biomedical tasks of a consultation would seem to make the family doctor's consulting life impossibly complicated. However, things are not as bad as all that.

- Consultations already have aims – it is just that the aims are often not fully visible and explicit.
- Aims can be used as tools in a consultation. For example, having explored the problems and outlined the possible management options, what is your patient's top priority? Once it has been identified, a record should be kept of this priority. Next time you meet, progress can be measured against this priority, whatever other things have happened in the mean time. *'Last time you said that your main problem was that you were not sleeping because of the pain. How are you sleeping now? Do you think things are better, worse, or just the same? Shall we continue with this treatment or choose another? You have tried three different types of painkillers. Which ones do you prefer?'*.
- A set of aims often covers more than one consultation. Whether there has been a response to treatment will only be apparent at the next consultation. It is a very secure feeling when you know what you are going to do next time, whatever the new information presented. You can also let your patient know what you intend if the treatment does not work. They will then know what to expect, and can be thinking about whether or not they will go along with it.

It is not practicable to achieve all of the possible aims in the same consultation. For example, an aim may not be realistic. Another aim may become less of a priority with time. A family doctor and her patient may agree to change the aims. This process of dodging and switching can go on for years, and may keep a family doctor and her patient going for a professional lifetime. Sometimes there are no aims left, and the family doctor does not know what to do next – this must be a pretty good definition of a 'heartsink' situation.[8]

Aim setting for depression

By way of an example, this section suggests how the idea of aims would deal with this common and potentially difficult problem in family practice. A presentation of depression is frequently the opener for a series of prolonged and possibly stressful consultations, often over a course of months or even years. The application of aims clarifies what is going on, and offers a framework of care from which everyone benefits.

First consultation

Possible patient aims
- I want these symptoms to improve.
- I want to feel more enthusiastic about my children, my job and my hobbies.
- I want a treatment that will mean I can cope with any side-effects.

Safety
- Stay alert to the risk of self-harm.

Possible clinical aims
- How certain is the diagnosis, and how often should it be reviewed?
- I need to establish and maintain a rapport so that the management plan can be implemented.
- The balance of benefits and side-effects of medication needs to remain explicit.
- Both I and my patient need to be committed to the management plan. What will alert me to the need for a change of plan?

Possible professional aims
- Reaching the diagnosis and the pursuit of the management plan should accord with best practice.
- I should be honest, trustworthy and able to keep a confidence.

Possible organisational aims
- This first consultation will almost certainly over-run the appointment time, but if the required work is done then this will save time later.
- Follow-up arrangements should be clinically appropriate, but also timed to try to avoid the need for emergency consultations.
- Information exchange with the team – either in the written record or verbally – must make the diagnosis and management plan easy to follow.

Possible personal aims
- I must not get overwhelmed by this patient's misery.
- I must be realistic about what can be achieved.
- Do I know what to do at the next consultation?
- Will I need a break before the next patient?

Subsequent consultations

If the first consultation has been conducted properly, the next one can be much more focused. In some cases, the first consultation has to be conducted in parts. A patient may be reluctant to disclose everything to you at a first meeting, either because of their illness or because they don't trust you – at least not yet. Other patients may remember things that they wanted to say only after the consultation has ended. Some will be surprised at what is happening and so more forgetful. However, once the information for the initial consultation has been gathered, either at one bite or in pieces, then the aims for subsequent consultations are different.

Possible patient aims

- In some respects I feel better, but there are some things I forgot to mention before – things which might lead to a more accurate diagnosis and treatment. Some of my symptoms are improved but are still not right, and others are no better.

Safety

- Review the risk of self-harm – it may be higher than before.

Possible clinical aims

- Review the diagnosis.
- Is the patient still convinced about the management plan? Has he been taking the medication as prescribed?
- I need to be sure that this consultation emphasises the positive. If this consultation is an action replay of the first, only dealing with what is still wrong, it will be difficult for a patient to achieve a more optimistic frame of mind. On the other hand, there may be vital information that is still outstanding.

Possible professional aims

- Am I maintaining my professional demeanour? Could this be interfering with communication and should it be relaxed?
- How much pressure is appropriate to encourage the patient to take his medication?

Possible organisational aims

- Is it safe to leave the rest until next time?
- When is a review appropriate?
- Are there already potentially difficult consultation(s) booked on the same day as the proposed review?
- Have there been any crisis consultations, and can these be avoided in future?

Possible personal aims

- How often can I cope with reviewing this problem?
- Am I sufficiently confident in this clinical area to want this patient to recommend me to his depressed friends?
- I want this patient and his family to appreciate the time and effort that I am expending on his care, but also to appreciate that I think he is worth it.

Summary

A consultation needs direction. Thinking in terms of aims rather than targets to define that direction makes more sense. There are many legitimate stakeholders in every consultation, and aims have to be framed to deal with all of the competing interests. It is neither possible nor reasonable to achieve more than four aims in a consultation, so long as patient safety has been secured – and then the consultation is 'good enough'. Aims can be shared and agreed with patients. Consultations already have aims, but they are often not explicit and transparent.

References

1. Freeman G, Carr J and Hill A (2004) The journey towards patient-centredness. *Br J Gen Pract.* **54**: 651–2.
2. Briscoe S (2005) *Britain in Numbers.* Politicos, London.
3. Zeithaml VA and Bitner MJ (1996) *Services Marketing.* McGraw-Hill International, Singapore.
4. Silverman J, Kurtz S and Draper J (2004) *Skills for Communicating with Patients* (2e). Radcliffe Publishing, Oxford.
5. Rawcliffe C (1997) *Medicine and Society in Later Medieval England.* Sutton Publishing, Stroud.
6. Neighbour R (1987) *The Inner Consultation.* Petroc, Newbury.
7. Bettelheim B (1987) *A Good Enough Parent.* Thames and Hudson, London.
8. Mathers NJ and Gask L (1995) Surviving the 'heartsink' experience. *Fam Pract.* **12**: 176–83.

Chapter 5

'R' is for room

The importance of spaces

As early as the eighteenth century, people were speculating that the physical environments within which healthcare was provided had an effect on the outcome. In the late nineteenth century Florence Nightingale suggested that:

> The first requirement of a hospital should be that it should do the sick no harm. *Notes on Hospitals*, 1859

She also pointed out that:

> The effect on sickness of beautiful objects, of variety of objects, and especially of brilliance of colours is hardly at all appreciated. . . . People say the effect is on the mind. It is no such thing. The effect is on the body, too. Little as we know about the way in which we are affected by form, by colour, by light, we do know this, that they have a physical effect. Variety of form and brilliancy of colour in the objects presented to patients is the actual means of recovery. *Notes on Hospitals*, 1859

This led to her advocacy of a particular size and arrangement for the individual hospital ward, still referred to as the 'Nightingale Ward'. It is a sign of her times that Florence Nightingale seems a little sniffy about the suggestion that the hospital environment should have an effect only on the mind of her patients, rather than on their physical state. Most designers of healthcare premises nowadays would be delighted if their building contributed in any way to the well-being of users.

There is continuing controversy about whether and by how much a physical environment can contribute to the mood, creativity or productivity of the people using it. Those in favour of the idea point to a sizeable body of research in their support. Others question the reliability of the research and highlight various confounding factors. For instance, the Hawthorne experiments in the 1920s showed that workers responded favourably when their working environment was changed in any respect, as if the benefit was gained from the novelty rather than from the form of the new environment. Critics refer to an assertion of the link between buildings and the minds of the people in them as *architectural determinism*.[1]

A number of studies have confirmed the physiological effects of environment, and reinforce the view that a 'therapeutic environment' is a realistic objective. The most influential features appear to be the following:

- light
- heat shielding

- humidity
- temperature
- music
- sound
- noise levels
- window views.[2]

Studies of the psychological effects of the healthcare environment confirm the importance of privacy and territoriality, and the fact that the arrangement of furniture in a room affects the way in which people behave and interact.[2]

The challenge for the BARD family doctor is to recognise that her surgery premises will almost certainly be having an effect on her patients. In addition, she must decide what effect she and her other workers are intending the surgery environment to have.

The physical environment of the surgery also has an effect on the family doctors and staff who spend most of their time and do most of their work there. The building should be functional – that is, fit for the purpose for which it is to be used. Using technology and engineering and construction techniques, the design of the surgery should be fully integrated, robust, smart and durable. The internal and external appearance should be pleasing and appropriate.[2] An additional consideration is that the surgery may well be owned by the family doctors, so they have an extra vested interest in striking a balance between usefulness and extravagance.

The building that a family doctor uses for her work will always be subject to compromise. If it has been converted, then there are the constraints of its existing bricks and mortar. If it has been purpose-built, then finance and any building or planning regulations must be considered. It is not possible to predict with accuracy what the future may bring with regard to how family doctor surgery premises are provided, but it is probably safe to assume that any options will not include the availability of unlimited financial resources.

The internal design of the building will be subject to the same constraints. Sometimes a family doctor will be able to lay claim to a consulting room for her use only, but often the inexorable expansion in primary care staff means that rooms are shared by other family doctors doing the same job, or by non-doctors who might be using the space for a variety of different jobs. Considerable research has been done on the design of rooms according to what is going to take place in them, so the architectural community acknowledges the value of designing rooms for tasks rather than for the particular individuals who will work in them.[2] A family doctor may feel that she wishes to personalise her consulting room and make it her own territory, but she should be aware that her architect probably thinks differently – there is a clear opportunity for creative compromise here.

Everyone will want a say in the design of communal spaces such as waiting rooms and reception areas.

A protected environment

For the family doctor, there are additional constraints on surgery and consulting-room design. Not only must the spaces be fit for their purpose, but also patients must feel safe and able to discuss the reasons why they have attended. The Introduction to this book discussed van Gannep's analysis of how social changes occur,[3] and how such ideas are also applicable to a family practice consultation. Three phases were identified. As far as a family practice consultation is concerned, *separation* is the phase in which a person wants something changed and decides to consult a doctor about it, *transition* is the consultation itself, when new ideas are generated to solve the problem, and *reincorporation* is the phase during which matters resolve to a new order of things. On the whole it is in the middle and last sections – *transition* and *reincorporation* – that family doctors ply their trade.

The process of *transition* in a family doctor consultation will nearly always cause anxiety. This is the phase when many new ideas are produced, where it is possible to 'think the unthinkable'. There must be no restriction on the ideas that a family doctor and her patient can throw into the pot for consideration, however unlikely they are. In fact, the more ideas that are considered, the more chance there is of choosing the right one. Some items on the agenda will cause anxiety because they are frightening. For example, in many consultations in primary care it is necessary to consider a diagnosis of cancer, not because it is particularly likely but because it is an important diagnosis not to miss. A good way to miss an important diagnosis is not to think of the possibility of its presence. Other agenda items cause anxiety just because they are new and different and do not accord with the normal familiar order of things. Such ideas must be aired in a place that is recognised both as being safe, and as being a location where such activities occur.

It is important that the family doctor understands the effect that coming to the surgery and engaging in a consultation is likely to have on her patients. A family doctor's surgery must be a place where her patients feel protected, where private and privileged information can be freely disclosed, and where anxiety-inducing topics such as illness, disability, death and suffering are talked about – topics that people would normally rather avoid discussing. The place in which this is done has to be separated from the rest of the world, so that the chaos and anxiety generated by the process of *transition* can be left behind there afterwards. There can then be a psychological as well as a physical leap from the real world into the world of illness, and a corresponding leap out again when normality (albeit slightly changed normality) is restored.

Reincorporation is the phase when a patient begins to come to terms with the new information offered and the changes that the future may bring. Like all adjustments, it takes time, but a start must be made during the consultation itself, to make sure that the patient is in a fit state to face the outside world. For some patients with some types of problem it is not possible to allow sufficient time for them to regain their public face. For those patients who feel unprepared to walk out through a waiting room, it is useful if the surgery has a back door.

It is the patient's perception of the appropriateness of the environment that is important. Notwithstanding the constraints of constructing a surgery in terms of function and design, a family doctor's surgery also has to appear to patients like a family doctor's surgery – that is, sufficiently reminiscent of other family doctor surgeries to feel familiar and safe. Patients know what to expect from a surgery, and will be bemused if there is much variation from this standard. Patients need to feel secure when consulting, otherwise the consultations will be less effective.

Entrance[5.1]

How can you encourage people to be in the right frame of mind as they enter your surgery?

- Are there visible signs to show where the surgery is?
- Are patients clearly shown where the front door is, either by means of signs or (better[2]) by the layout of the building?
- There could be railings or shutters, depending on security needs. Are the doors glass or solid? If they are made of glass, is it frosted, smoked or clear? What can a patient see when they look through the glass?
- Should there be a pram park?
- Should cyclists be encouraged by providing a secure parking area specifically for them?
- What is the parking provision like? Presumably the family doctor will want to encourage as many patients as possible to attend the surgery rather than request home visits. Is there any provision for 'disabled' parking?
- Where are the bus-stops? Could the bus companies be encouraged to site them more conveniently?

Waiting rooms

Many patients spend more time in the waiting room than they do in the consulting room, and while they are there they will probably have more than enough time to look at their environment. Although the waiting-room environment is probably not as important to the overall experience of 'going to the doctor's' as other factors (e.g. the family doctor's communication skills), it nevertheless has some impact. Patients will inevitably interpret the waiting room as representative of their family doctor's attitude towards them.

- Are the waiting areas comfortable, clean and properly heated?
- Is there adequate space to cope with the potential throughput of patients?
- Are there enough chairs? Are the chairs too low and lacking arms so that the infirm are unable to get in and out of them, and so more likely to request a home visit next time? Are the chairs comfortable, relatively new and in good repair? If not, what does this say about what the family doctor thinks of her patients?
- What is on the noticeboards? It would be easy to completely cover the walls with health education posters, notices about voluntary groups, pleas about the use of the emergency services, and imperfectly crayoned invitations to the church bazaar. Should the local school be asked to lend you some of the children's work for display? Does the family practice have a policy about putting up posters for local groups or businesses?
- Is there reading material available? If it is health related, have the contents been checked both for accuracy and for accordance with practice attitudes and policies?

[5.1] Is it a coincidence that 'entrance' meaning the door to a building is the same word as 'entrance' as in 'cast a spell'?

- Is there a means of keeping small children amused so that they do not run around and disturb other patients?
- What about music? If there are problems with sound insulation, having background music may be a way of ensuring confidentiality. Even if the sound permeates the consulting rooms, most people find it relaxing and think that it makes a positive contribution to the consultation.[4]
- What is access to the reception desk like? Can patients in the waiting area overhear conversations at the desk? Is there a separate area for patients who do not want their requests to be broadcast around their neighbours? Can telephone conversations be overheard from the waiting room? What can be seen of activity in the reception area from the waiting room?

> John's new practice had two sites, so all of the consulting rooms were used by more than one doctor. John could not help noticing that at one site the most senior partner consulting at each session would always insist on using a particular room, even if this meant moving all the papers and clutter from the previous session. The popular room was called 'Room 1', and it was nearest to the waiting room. Furthermore, in the waiting room was a list of the doctors consulting at that session, and the occupant of Room 1 was always at the top of the list.

Violence

Violence towards family doctors and other primary care staff is a significant and worsening problem. A survey of family doctors in Leeds in the UK showed that over a 12-month period 54% had been subjected to verbal abuse, 28% had received specific threats, 6% had been subject to physical attack and in just under 2% of cases the attack was with a weapon or led to physical injury.[5] Fortunately, although threats are common, actual attacks resulting in injury are rare. There is little information available about violence towards primary care reception and nursing staff.[6]

Primary care surgery buildings can be designed to minimise the occurrence and adverse effects of violent activity. A solution to the potentially conflicting demands of ease of access, confidentiality and safety should be found. Possible solutions might include the following.

- Ensure that all of the waiting space can be observed from the reception area.
- Avoid the use of barriers, grilles and glass screens.
- Ensure that staff have a way of leaving the reception area which does not involve going through the waiting area.[6]

Specific suggestions for minimising risk in waiting rooms include the following.

- Paint the walls in pastel colours.
- Keep patients informed, especially about delays.
- Install a payphone.
- Have clean, well-signposted toilets available.
- Provide access to a cold drinks dispenser.

- Provide appropriate entertainment in the form of reading material, music and/ or television.
- Ideally the room should have windows, preferably looking out on a natural scene or a landscaped garden with a fountain. If the room has no windows, then a *trompe-l'oeil* picture designed to look like a view from a window is better than nothing.
- If there is artwork on the walls, it should be of good quality.
- The reception desk should preferably project into the waiting area so that there is good all-round visibility. The counter should be 1200 mm high and 800 mm deep – this makes physical violence nearly impossible without seeming to be too much of a physical or auditory barrier.
- Waiting-room chairs can be set as outurned circles or ovals, so that patients are not staring at each other, but can talk to their neighbours if they wish.
- Have panic buttons available for staff.

When John joined the practice, he wondered why one waiting area was so large that it had an echo and made patients nervous, while the other was so small that patients frequently spilled into the corridor. The partners responsible for planning the building had, in their wisdom, decided that a large waiting room would be ideal for community events and public meetings. In the 10 years since construction there had been two public meetings and three staff parties in that room. A change in the surgery rota meant that all of the consulting rooms adjacent to the small waiting area were often in use at the same time.

Consulting rooms

According to feng shui, the flow of *sheng qi* (i.e. the good, positive universal energy) should be encouraged by giving due regard to the interplay of rooms and furniture.[7] Whether you accept the validity of feng shui or not, it is undeniable that the configuration of rooms and the type and position of furniture have a demonstrable psychological effect,[2] so it makes sense to ensure that this effect is as beneficial as possible.

- How big is the room? A large room with a high ceiling can be daunting, and suggests that the family doctor is pompous. On the other hand, the room must be large enough to contain the necessary furniture and equipment.
- The lighting must be adequate, but must it always be harsh and fluorescent? What would softer lighting say about how the family doctor wants the consultation to proceed?
- Which way does the door open? Should the contents of the room be revealed each time the door is opened, or should the door open the other way, making a barrier for the patient to negotiate?
- What wheelchair access is available both into the building and around the building? If healthcare professionals cannot be thoughtful enough to make adequate provision for disability, what hope is there for the disabled patient in other buildings that they may visit?

- Where are the windows? How large are they? Plenty of natural light will tend to soften the effect of the overall lighting, but large windows can mean that the room gets uncomfortably hot on sunny days. Who can overlook the windows? Do they provide adequate privacy and also security?
- What about the decorating? Cool *yin* colours such as blues and greens are supposed to induce calm and be beneficial to thinking and reading,[7] and they are also quite pleasant colours.
- Are there pictures on the walls? A few landscapes will offer some compensation if nothing much can be seen out of the windows. Alternatively, patients could be invited to lend their own work for display. It is surprising how much talent there is out there, and the patients will usually play the game by only offering their best efforts. Certificates of medical qualifications may on the one hand indicate expertise, but on the other may appear pretentious. Certificates sited behind the family doctor's chair will be a distraction. Spoof certificates (e.g. 'The World's Messiest Drinker') should only be displayed by family doctors who feel that they want to offer a flippant self-image to every patient who consults with them.
- Many family doctors have personal items, such as photographs of their children, in their consulting room. To a family doctor who spends most of her working life in that room, such personal touches make it a little more homely. They also indicate to patients 'I am a normal person with a normal family and normal wants in life.' Yet there is a downside. Many patients will be attending because they are (or feel) deprived of the normality which the family doctor's decorations confirm that she has achieved. Patients may not want to think of the surgery as anything other than a streamlined and efficient health factory. And they may also be prompted to ask you about your children – in which case what are you prepared to tell them?

> The surgery was a modern building with lots of straight lines and right angles, but John thought that the door to the staff toilet was set at an uncharacteristically peculiar angle. He found out that it was set like this so that the door could not be seen from the waiting room, as the doctors were embarrassed by patients in the waiting room seeing them going to use the toilet.

Furniture

Furniture can be moved around to a limited extent, subject of course to the overall room layout and the position of the plugs and phone terminals. Sometimes it is worth moving things about just to make a change,[1] and a family doctor will often intuitively hit on an arrangement that seems right. However, she must also be mindful of the impression that this is creating.

If the family doctor has her back to a window, on sunny days her patients will not be able to see her face, and her head will be surrounded by an angelic glow. Lip-readers will have no chance of finding out what she is saying. Similarly, if her desk faces the door, patients entering the room will be confronted by a barrier, and they will also be right in the doctor's field of view all the time. This can be unnerving, so set the desk at an angle or to one side.

Large executive-style chairs that swivel round will emphasise a family doctor's sense of self-importance. Is her chair larger and/or higher than that of her patient? What does this say about her and her attitude towards her patients? Is she literally looking down on them? Is this the impression that should be created? Chairs need arms so that the family doctor can lean back and to one side (a sign of benevolent relaxation) without falling on the floor.[8]

Consulting across the corner of the desk suggests an atmosphere of trust and support.[8] If there is nothing at all between the family doctor and the patient, some patients will react by feeling threatened and behaving defensively. Right-handed doctors should probably have the patient at the left side of the desk so that the writing hand is on the desk side.

Four *spatial zones* have been identified which indicate how comfortable people are likely to be with others nearby.

- The *public zone* has a 4-metre radius, and applies at public events such as lectures or shows. People are uneasy if the players encroach nearer than this.
- The *social zone* has a radius of between 1.25 and 4 metres, and this kind of space makes people who are acquaintances feel at ease.
- The *personal zone* has a radius of 0.5 to 1.25 metres, and applies to people at social gatherings such as drinks parties who know each other well.
- The *intimate zone* is usually occupied only by partners and children. Doctors can be admitted temporarily to the intimate zone for the purposes of physical examination. Being close to the family doctor may be necessary for the fulfilment of the work of the consultation, but many patients will find it uncomfortable.

A computer screen in a consulting room could never be described as discreet and, just like the family television, it inevitably becomes the focus of the room. The screen is best sited so that both the family doctor and the patient can see it, but this also means that a family doctor who is looking at the screen cannot at the same time be looking at her patient. The best compromise is to leave only the screen, keyboard and mouse on the desk, and (assuming that the family doctor is consulting over the corner of the desk) to site the screen at the end of the desk furthest from the patient. A computer screen can be used as a barrier to communication, but then so can paper records if that is what the family doctor wishes.

An examination couch and attendant light source are quite bulky items, and cannot be easily hidden away. Their presence is a reminder that although the consulting room is primarily set up for conversation, there is always the possibility that a clinical examination will be required. During the talking part of a consultation, the family doctor and the patient are on roughly equal terms. A clinical examination is very much the family doctor's preserve, and she is very obviously in charge. Just what is she feeling for? Will it hurt? Will her hands be cold? What can she hear with those pipes in her ears? The skills of examination are a closed book to most patients, so the mysterious quality of medical practice is very prominent during examination. This is probably why examination is so highly prized by patients ('I just want you to listen to my chest'), especially if it involves instruments, even though in most cases a clinical examination is unlikely to alter a management decision.[9] Although the presence of a couch may encourage more physical examinations, it will only be used for a minority of consultations. However, its presence has an invasive effect on all consultations.

An examination often requires the removal of clothing, and most people do not feel at their most confident when partially dressed. What if the consulting room door is opened, revealing the examinee to the occupants of the waiting room?

Some equipment, such as a stethoscope, sphygmomanometer and auriscope, should be readily available for all consultations. Other items will only be used occasionally. Items that go out of date, such as syringes and needles, are better stored separately – someone reliable (i.e. not a family doctor) can be charged with keeping the stock up to date. If clinical equipment is readily to hand, it is more likely to be used. Owing to the nature of the job, most items of clinical equipment will only be used very rarely by a family doctor, so it is not inevitable that they will be used properly. Will the proximity of such equipment encourage incompetence? Medical accoutrements left on view to patients will, rather like the dentist's drill, leave an impression that may not be the one intended.

Dress

Patients do notice how their family doctor is dressed, and their perceptions leave impressions which may affect consultation outcomes. Most work in this area has been done with hospital doctors and patients. Children in Birmingham in the UK regard formally dressed paediatricians as competent but not friendly, and casually dressed paediatricians as friendly but not competent.[10] In Israel, medical patients prefer their physician to wear a white coat (especially if the physician is older), and semi-formal clothing otherwise. They do not like long hair, earrings and sandals on male physicians and short skirts, shorts and tight clothes on female physicians. However, 75% of patients in the same survey said that clothing would not affect their choice of family doctor.[11] Australian patients also prefer formal attire and feel that it inspires confidence and trust – and are opposed to nose rings.[12]

> John was clear that he made a priority of emphasising the empathic aspect of his professional role. Accordingly he decided on a relaxed and friendly style of consulting, but one that was technically competent. He wanted to wear jeans to work. However, there were raised eyebrows among the other family doctors he worked with (which he was rather proud about), but also mutterings from his elderly patients. He eventually reverted to a collar and tie but definitely no suit and no white coat.

In a rare survey from primary care, Scottish patients were found to favour male family doctors in a formal suit, and female doctors in a white coat. A male doctor in a tweed jacket and informal shirt and tie was least disliked. A quarter of the patients said that they would be unhappy consulting with an informally dressed family doctor, and two-thirds felt that the way a family doctor dresses is either important or very important.[13]

John's own family doctor trainer was a dapper chap with three generations of authority as the village family doctor. On home visits, in winter or summer, he would wear a trilby hat which looked several sizes too small. It was such an obvious affectation, and quite at variance with his other clothes.

One day, when he felt confident enough to pass comment, John asked his trainer why he wore the hat. *'It is so that I can take it off when I go into a house, and put it on again when I am going to leave,'* he replied.

Doubtless patients regard the personality of a family doctor as more important than her appearance, but it nevertheless makes sense to be aware of all the factors that might be affecting consultations and patient care. Patients want to see a family doctor who looks like a family doctor, and so are perplexed when she looks different, even if the intention is to create a more understanding image. A family doctor who adopts a casual and thoughtless approach to her attire may be thought to take an equally slipshod approach to her work.

Clothes have to be practical for the job. Colours that need frequent cleaning are less suitable, and there need to be sufficient pockets. Any jewellery must be chosen so as not to interfere with the job or scratch the patients.

Using the spaces

Just speak up, and try and miss the furniture.
Noel Coward

Most consultations are conducted with the family doctor and the patient both seated. Why should this be? Is there anything to be gained by standing up and walking about on occasion, in order to employ a fuller repertoire of body movements?

- A family doctor might walk to the door and greet her patient. A shake of the hand may be offered. These are pieces of anachronistic courteous nonsense, but they are unlikely to cause offence and will be welcomed by many patients.
- Standing up and moving punctuates the consultation. One piece of the business is over, and the next is starting. A family doctor might try standing up when she has heard enough, or when she thinks that it's time that she said something.
- Standing and walking towards a patient implies that an examination is about to take place. Clinical examination is highly rated by most patients, and gives the family doctor the chance to look impressive by doing things which most people cannot do.
- A separate examination room is often useful. Pelvic and rectal examinations are somehow more seemly if conducted in a separate room, and a chaperone can be more easily called if needed to assist. If the family doctor is really pressed, she can also be seeing another patient while the examinee is preparing for the examination.

- Help the patient on with his coat.
- Hold the door open when the patient is leaving (or when you want him to leave).
- It also does a family doctor no harm to stretch her legs or even leave the consulting room during a surgery. Such breaks should not be prolonged, especially if the surgery is over-running (which, ironically, is when a family doctor is most likely to want a break). It is usually possible for a family doctor to look earnest and create the impression to the waiting room that she has been called out to an emergency in another part of the building, or to an urgent phone call.

Summary

The place where consultations take place has an effect on those consultations. Surgery premises must be fit for their purpose for both the family doctor and the patient. For the doctor this means that the premises must be functional and efficient, and economical to build and maintain. For the patient this means that the premises must be comfortable and businesslike, and must also look as a surgery is supposed to look if the patient is to feel safe to transact the anxious business that a consultation usually involves.

References

1. Marmot A (2002) Architectural determinism. *Br J Gen Pract.* **52**: 252–3.
2. Francis S (2002) The architecture of health buildings. *Br J Gen Pract.* **52**: 254–5.
3. van Gannep A (1960) *The Rites of Passage* (trans. MB Vizedon and GL Caffee). Chicago University Press, Chicago.
4. Kabler JJ (1993) Background music in consultations (letter). *Br J Gen Pract.* **43**: 172.
5. Ness GJ, House A and Ness AR (2000) Aggression and violent behaviour in general practice: population-based survey in the north of England. *BMJ.* **320**: 1447–8.
6. Wright NMJ, Dixon CAJ and Tompkins CNE (2003) Managing violence in primary care: an evidence-based approach. *Br J Gen Pract.* **53**: 557–62.
7. Henwood B (1997) *Feng Shui.* Parkgate Books, London.
8. Wainwright GR (2003) *Teach Yourself Body Language.* Hodder & Stoughton, London.
9. Tate P (1997) *The Doctor's Communication Handbook* (2e). Radcliffe Medical Press, Oxford.
10. Barrett TG and Booth IW (1994) Sartorial eloquence: does it exist in the paediatrician–patient relationship? *BMJ.* **309**: 1710–12.
11. Menahem S and Shvartzman P (1998) Is our appearance important to our patients? *Fam Pract.* **15**: 391–7.
12. Nair BR, Attia JR, Mears SR *et al.* (2002) Evidence-based physician's dressing: a crossover trial. *Med J Aust.* **177**: 681–2.
13. McKinstry B and Wang JX (1991) Putting on the style: what patients think of the way their doctor dresses. *Br J Gen Pract.* **41**: 275–8.

Chapter 6

'D' is for dialogue

'When I *use a word,'* Humpty Dumpty said in a rather scornful tone, *'it means just what I choose it to mean – neither more nor less.'*

Lewis Carroll, *Through the Looking-Glass*

Successful communication is achieved when what is in the brain of the speaker is matched by what is in the brain of the listener. Transmission and reception are both important, but it is what appears in the consciousness of the receiver that is of paramount importance. To this end, the participants in a consultation must at least be speaking the same language. Words that are not understood are worse than useless – not only is no meaning imparted, but also consternation and confusion are caused. Consulting like Humpty Dumpty is not a valid option for a family doctor who takes her job and profession seriously.

Less than 10% of communication is determined by the words being used.[1] Nevertheless, a person will speak around 40 000 words in a day, nearly 90% of which are about personal relationships and experiences – love lives, TV programmes and jokes.[2] If there is conflict between the words and the non-verbal messages, the body language usually wins,[3] but conflict is also likely to result in confusion for the listener. For maximum effect and optimum communication to be achieved, the body language and the words should be giving the same message.

For both of these reasons it is important for the family doctor to give some thought to the words she will use in a consultation – to make sure that she and her patient are on the same wavelength, and to reinforce the rest of her behaviour.

Preconceptions

In general terms, people hear most readily what they are expecting to hear. If something unexpected is communicated, then there is a need not only to assimilate the new information, but also to cope with the reason why the listener's expectations have not been realised. A family doctor who wishes to optimise her verbal communication must be aware of her patients' preconceptions.

There are a number of reasons why family doctors and their patients think about health in different ways, resulting in possible confusion and miscommunication. The general standard of medical knowledge in the community is poor.[4] This is not to say that people do not have knowledge that they regard as being medically correct. Just the reverse. There is a lot of knowledge about illness and medicine out there, but much of it is wrong.

- People are on the whole logical. They will try and make sense of their illnesses with the knowledge that they have available. These rationalisations for illness have been termed *explanatory models*.[5] They are frequently shared within the patient's social circle, and include knowledge from various sources, including science, religion and anecdote. Such explanatory models are truly believed, and will often pass down the generations.

- Sometimes a term is used to explain an illness pattern, but it has no apparent scientific basis. What exactly is a 'chill' or a 'nervous breakdown'? Such *folk illness* is found all over the world, and is especially prevalent in places without a scientific healthcare tradition.[5]
- The *locus of control* model[4] suggests that some people feel that their health is controlled by their own efforts (internal locus of control), while others think that the causes of illness are external and so cannot be altered (external locus of control). This explains why some people are prepared to make changes to their lifestyle in order to improve their health, and others are not. Health information that does not accord with a patient's locus of control is unlikely to be agreed with.
- People also show distinct preferences for the categories of health information that they want to hear. These preferences for information, in order of priority, are as follows:[6]
  - diagnosis
  - prognosis
  - aetiology and prevention
  - treatment
  - social effects ('Can I visit my grandchildren?', 'Can I have a drink?').

Patients from all social classes express a clear desire to be well informed about their health. Unfortunately, patients from more deprived social classes (or who their family doctor believes are from these classes) are offered fewer relevant explanations about their condition and treatment.[4]

The best way to find out about a person's health beliefs is to ask them. It is tempting for a family doctor to be clever and try to predict what a patient believes about their symptoms, but the likelihood of being wrong is very high. Then all the family doctor has is a bemused patient who has no idea what she is talking about, but who will often not say anything for fear of appearing foolish. As a result the family doctor will never find out what is really on her patient's mind.

John, like the great communicator he hoped to be, was talking to an ex-miner who had just had a heart attack. John explained how the rest of this patient's heart muscle would, in time, get stronger in compensation for the part that had been damaged during the attack.

The next week John's patient returned and said: *'I've been thinking about what you said, and I've decided that if it works we can share the money.'* It appeared that the previous week it was the word 'compensation' which had left the deepest impression.

Transmitting and receiving

Verbal information has to be transmitted from the mind of the family doctor to the mind of the patient, and vice versa. The family doctor is the professional, and she has a duty to do as much as possible to ensure the success of the communication. The stages of verbal communication – thoughts into words, words into speech, speech received, speech interpreted as intended – can all be influenced by improving technique. Conversely, it is the family doctor who has the professional responsibility for interpreting correctly what a patient says.

Hearing

Can your patient hear what is being said? This may sound like a trivial point, but it can make a lot of difference to a consultation, especially if the content of what is being said is unexpected and so needs some thought. Some of the hard of hearing cope by unconsciously lip-reading, but they can't do this if their family doctor is not looking at them, or has her hand over her mouth. Users of hearing aids will often switch them off in public places, such as the waiting room, because many different sources of noise are confusing, and they may subsequently forget to switch them on again.

Quantity

Patients forget up to 80% of the things that their family doctor tells them,[7] and they have a preference for retaining the things that they want to hear. A patient who is presented with a piece of bad news will nearly always not be listening to what he is told next. Important information, such as the treatment plan, has to be discussed there and then. If there is a lot of information to share, then the less urgent parts can be let out more gradually, and possibly over several sittings.

   As well as hearing what he wants to hear, a patient is also more likely to remember the information that he wants to know. One way of finding out what a patient wants to know is to wait until he asks specific questions. However, this does run the risk of the family doctor appearing reluctant to offer information, or of failing because a shy patient will not ask questions. The use of a comment such as 'Is there anything you want to ask me about?' can be of value.

Be specific

As was grudgingly conceded in Chapter 4 on aims, there are a number of limited occasions when targets can be useful in a consultation. The more concrete the advice that a patient is offered, the more memorable it will be to him. Many family doctors are reluctant to give specific advice because they know the limitations of the precepts upon which that advice is founded, and they do not like to be proved wrong. It is never certain that a particular patient is going to respond as the research predicts. However, a phrase such as 'It might help if you lost some weight' is less memorable than 'Follow this diet sheet. You will lose a stone by Christmas and your knees won't hurt any more'. The family doctor may feel a bit silly if by Christmas the promised improvement has not occurred, but on the other hand being specific will probably have resulted in some progress.

Perhaps coping with feeling silly should be added to the list of professional qualities required by a family doctor.

Time

If there is a lot of information to relay, don't try and give it all out at once. Decide what is most important, and make arrangements for a further interview to cover the rest. There will be some instances where this is impossible. If urgent decisions are needed, then it is important that the patient is sufficiently well informed to make those decisions. In this case, what is said should be paced. Pauses between pieces of information will allow it time to sink in. Questions may be asked to make sure that the main pieces of information have been understood. This all takes time, but better an over-running surgery than a patient who is rushed into a decision that they later regret.

Primacy and explicit categorisation

When offering information to a patient, what is said first is more likely to be remembered than what is said subsequently – this is known as the *primacy effect.*[4] It may be possible to present what the family doctor considers to be the most important information at the outset. She may, quite reasonably, want her patient to remember what treatment or lifestyle adjustments are needed, whereas her patient is more likely to want to know the diagnosis and prognosis. Key information can be conveyed more effectively by repeating it, several times if necessary. Using the technique of *explicit categorisation,*[8] everything is said three times – say what is going to be said, say it, and then summarise what has been said.

Social conversation

Patients are generally pleased if there is a little social chat in the consultation.[3] Some offers of such social engagement will be initiated by the patient, and the family doctor should have an idea beforehand of how much personal information she is prepared to share. Refusing to engage may well be seen by her patient as blocking the closeness of the interaction, whereas the family doctor may see it as maintaining a professional relationship.

The type of social information that the family doctor is prepared to share with her patients should also be given some thought. Ordinary areas of family and domestic life (e.g. 'How old are the children and what are they doing?', 'Did you see the football last night?') are relatively safe ground, but are also the areas where a family doctor may be most keen to protect her privacy. Areas to be avoided are issues of contention (e.g. politics, religion), and anything which may highlight the fact that family doctors and their patients in general have different lifestyles (e.g. where she went on holiday).

John did not want to seem aloof from any of his patients. He had watched his trainer address a few select patients by their first name, but they always called him 'Doctor Smith'. This sounded patronising, but still most of his own patients seemed happier to call him 'Doctor' as well. John eventually resolved to call everyone over the age of 18 by their title – 'Mr' or 'Mrs' or even 'sir'. On the few occasions that it happened, John was convinced that when a patient called him by his first name it made a difference to how the consultation went along.

The relationships that are built up through consultations have a therapeutic effect. However, a family doctor will not interact socially with her patients in the same way as she will with other people, though this is as it should be since the aims of the interaction are different. This is a consultation – not a cocktail party. The people who a family doctor is trained to treat are those with whom she has a professional relationship. She is unlikely to do an adequate job on people who she knows only outside her professional context.

How fast to speak?

If a family doctor speaks too fast, then she will be harder to hear, and there will be fewer opportunities for her patient to interrupt in order to obtain clarification. She will also sound as if she is nervous. On the other hand, the business of the consultation is transacted more quickly. A family doctor who speaks too slowly will run the risk of sounding patronising. As a rule of thumb, the family doctor should try and speak to her patients in complete sentences, and should pace her speech so that she knows when she starts a sentence how she intends to finish it.

How loud to speak?

The family doctor's voice should be loud enough to be heard, but not so loud that she sounds strident, and not so loud that the waiting room can join in with the consultation. If there is background noise or if the consultation is with a deaf patient, then a slight raising of the volume is inevitable. However, there are other tricks that can help with voice clarity. Lessons can be learned from actors who do television and radio work. It is not the volume of sound which makes the voice intelligible – it is the amount of breath that supports it. This technique also avoids the risk of voice strain (*see* Chapter 7 on training).

Around 50% of people over the age of 60 years have some impairment of their hearing. The Royal National Institute for the Deaf makes the following recommendations.[9]

- Ask your patient how they prefer to communicate.
- Ensure that the immediate environment is as quiet as possible.
- Stand or sit as close as is polite.
- Face your patient so that lip-reading is possible.
- Face the light so that your patient can see your lips and body language.
- Speak clearly with a normal rhythm.
- Do not shout.
- Avoid jargon and unfamiliar abbreviations.
- Sentences and phrases are easier to understand than single words. Try different words with the same meaning, or write it down.

- Keep hands, pens, etc. away from your mouth when speaking.
- Do not carry on talking if your face is turned away.
- Check that understanding has occurred.

> John was not at all sure that he liked Monica. She was always bad-tempered, and seemed to relish blaming anyone and everyone for her increasing disabilities. During one home visit, John asked her if she was having any problems with her hearing. *'Of course, I have got a hearing aid,'* she said, *'but I don't wear it because I don't need it. I can hear everything you say, you know.'* Talking later to Monica's long-suffering daughter, John asked if the hearing aid could be found and Monica encouraged to use it more. *'Oh no,'* came the reply. *'She doesn't like it, and anyway if she puts it in she can hear what we are saying about her.'*

What tone of voice?

Different situations require different modes of voice delivery. In most cases a confident, almost cheerful tone is best. *'Everything is under control. There is nothing to worry about. I've seen your sort of problem lots of times before, and I am confident that my proposed treatment will get you right.'* However, such an approach is certainly not appropriate for discussing, say, depression or the possibility of a termination of pregnancy, or for bereavement work. A family doctor's tone of voice will naturally reflect her frame of mind and her perception of any cues in the consultation. If a family doctor is in an appropriate role, then her tone of voice will also be appropriate.

The right words

After even a brief career, all family doctors find that the same situations keep recurring with different patients. A form of words may have been used in the past which appears to express very well what the family doctor wishes to communicate, and appears to be well received by patients. That sentence or phrase will be stored in the memory for future use.

With experience more and more such phrases will be stored up, tempting the family doctor to use familiar phrases either too much or too little. She may want to insert a stock phrase or two into a consultation where they just do not fit in properly. Alternatively, she may get so bored with repeating the same phrase time after time that she is tempted to say something different just for the novelty of it.

Communication feels at its most natural if it is (or appears to be) spontaneous. However, being spontaneous is not the same as being innovative. Being spontaneous is finding the right words at the right time, even if those words have been used a thousand times previously. A family doctor must also on occasion be innovative – that is, able to find new ways of expressing a thought. Innovation will be needed if the situation is genuinely novel, or if a previously tried and tested expression has not been understood or well received.

Family doctors often have a problem being innovative. You do not pass science exams by inventing facts. People who end up as family doctors have proved themselves able to accept the truth as delivered by others – whether the eminent professor or the randomised controlled trial. The idea of being innovative may not just be alien – it may be considered positively subversive.

Jargon

It has been suggested that the new words that are learned during medical undergraduate training amount to the equivalent of at least two foreign languages.[10] It is probably true that medical students learn more new words than anything else during their training. The dictionary definition of 'jargon' is illuminating:

> Unintelligible words, gibberish; barbarous or debased language; mode of speech full of unfamiliar terms; twittering of birds.[11]

Some medical words apply to important ideas and concepts, and as such are useful communication tools. Other words refer to things that are not and probably never will be widely discussed among the laity. These too are useful. However, there cannot be any justification for inventing a word for medical use when there is a perfectly good English equivalent. What exactly is the difference between a fractured bone and a broken bone? Or between a tibia and a shin bone? Or between coagulation and clotting? The medical words are invariably longer, harder to remember, and if their derivation has any logic it is dependent on a knowledge of classical languages.

In addition, medicine has hijacked a number of normal words and given them a different meaning. The medical and lay uses of the words 'hysterical' and 'chronic' are quite different. To most people (including, presumably, Alfred Hitchcock) 'vertigo' is a fear of heights, an understanding that would not be shared by an ear, nose and throat specialist, who would think of vertigo as a sensation of rotation. No doubt a fear of heights can cause a sensation of rotation, but nevertheless the word retains two distinct meanings. Communication can only succeed when the family doctor and the patient share the same under-standing of the words being used.

The use of acronyms when talking with patients is rarely if ever justified. Even those patients who are vaguely familiar with the acronym will need to pause to be sure that they are interpreting it correctly, and then what is said next is lost. Medical English and real English also have a slightly different grammar, even if the vocabulary is being understood.

Local words

In her laudable quest to make herself more intelligible to her patients the family doctor may, if she is not careful, be induced to use words and phrases that do not derive from her vocabulary of origin. This is nearly always a mistake, since it usually sounds utterly false. Similarly, getting an accent right needs enormous practice. The use of local words and phrases, except when quoting back some-thing that a patient has said, sounds equally phoney. Furthermore, it is not at all certain that the patient will welcome his family doctor's attempt to speak his own language in quite that way. Understanding the words that patients use is of vital importance, just as is understanding the beliefs that give rise to what is said.

However, patients expect their family doctor to speak a little differently – it's all part of the role.

> John had moved area with each step of his medical career, and despite being in the same family practice for 10 years, had never really come to terms with the local vernacular. When he first heard a patient say *'I'm not satisfied'*, he bristled with indignation and considered phoning his professional indemnity insurers. Only later did he realise that when a patient was 'not satisfied' this was not usually associated with an aggressive tone of voice. It eventually dawned on John that *'I'm not satisfied'* actually meant *'I'm still worried'* and not *'I intend to complain about you.'*

Expectations

There is a rider to all of this. Patients prefer their diagnosis to be expressed in medical rather than real words. Having a grand-sounding word for a diagnosis means that the symptoms have been taken seriously, that there is a definite cause for the illness, and that a period of incapacity is justified. This leads to increased patient satisfaction. On the other hand, the use of lay terms in diagnosis makes patients feel that their problem is trivial, and that it needs no medical input to solve it. It also implies that the patient has brought the illness on himself.[12]

> Although only in early middle age, Ann had for many years endured faecal incontinence, a problem not made easier by her preference for light-coloured clothing. Through all of this she retained a cheerfulness and healthy distrust of the efforts of her medical advisers. John suggested to her that a bout of vague but troublesome symptoms had been caused by a viral infection.
>
> At their next meeting Ann told John that she understood that he had no idea why her symptoms had been so bad. This perplexed John, who again stated his opinion that a virus had caused the problem. *'Oh really?'*, replied Ann, *'I thought doctors only said things were due to a virus when they did not know the real reason.'*

The idea that names are important is very ancient, and it is a feature of many communities. The entity and the name may come to be the same thing. In cultures where magic is or was important, it can often be done using the name just as readily as it can be done by having possession of the entity.[13] The fact that patients in the developed countries where magic is not usually a fact of life still like to have their symptoms subjected to a label (a diagnosis), and that they prefer that label to be given in a foreign and ancient language, hints at an enduring link with the healers/magicians of the past.

Representation system

Neurolinguistic programming suggests that people are of four types with respect to their preferences for verbal communication. These 'sublanguages' or 'representational systems' affect the way in which they use and receive language. The preferred type is reflected in the words used.

For instance, if a patient is a 'visual' type then he will use words like 'see', 'appear' and 'show'. He will also be more understanding of words if they are also of a 'visual' nature. Those with an 'auditory' preference respond to words like 'hear', 'sound' and 'listen'. 'Kinaesthenic' types respond to words like 'touch', 'feel' and 'grasp'. The fourth group are the 'audiodigitals', a small group who tend to have conversations with themselves. It is often possible to pick up from a patient what type he is by listening specifically to the words that he uses. If the same words or types of words are used in return by the family doctor, communication is likely to be more effective.[1]

Misinterpretation

Patients prefer to be asked about their 'concerns' rather than their 'worries'.[3] The word 'worry' implies a neurotic reaction to a benign situation, whereas 'concern' is a perfectly reasonable response to dangerous events.

Family doctors use the pronoun 'we' in consultations far more than patients do. They may use the word inclusively, so that 'we' means 'me and you'. However, many patients interpret the 'we' exclusively, as in 'we in the medical profession'. Similarly, on the rare occasions when patients use the pronoun 'we', it usually refers to the patient's family, and does not include the family doctor. It is suggested that family doctors should use 'I', 'you' and 'me', in order to avoid misunderstanding.[14]

'Let's see what happens' and 'I don't know' have been identified by patients as phrases used by family doctors which are particularly detrimental to inspiring confidence.[15] Involving patients in the uncertainty of decision making in primary care may be a very laudable attempt at sustaining the ethical principle of autonomy, so long as the result is the one intended.

In 75% of cases when a patient laughs during a consultation he gets no response at all from his family doctor. Laughter is seen as an invitation to 'come closer', and there will be problems if the offer is not reciprocated. Failure to join in the laughter may be interpreted as rejection or even as an expression of malice on the part of the family doctor.[16]

Creativity

The most memorable and effective communication is that which is apparently unique and personalised. An exchange of monologues is not good enough. A communication becomes special when the parties involved feel that their interaction has created something extra – something more than the sum of the parts. When creativity is apparent, the family doctor and the patient are responding to each other. A level of attention and concentration is being used that elevates the communication above the simply mechanical, and a closeness is generated. There are relationship as well as technical healthcare benefits when there is creativity. Patients and family doctors in a consultation both have an interest in making sure that the interaction is as creative as possible.

True dialogue can be achieved with good consultation techniques, responding to cues and clues, and by a family doctor who manages to make her patient feel (for his allotted time) as if he is the centre of the universe. However, a consultation is much more likely to feel unique if creativity has genuinely resulted.

If the best consultations have an element of creativity, is it possible to make yourself more creative? Acting teachers encourage creativity by the use of *improvisation*. Improvisation games are those in which learners are put into new and often bizarre situations. The outcome of the situation does not matter, so there can be no overall aim. The best improvisers are those who metaphorically 'walk into a room backwards'[17] – they are aware of where they have been but do not care where they are going. Examples of improvisations can be found in Chapter 7 on training. A family doctor who allows herself to be creative will see all the possibilities in a situation and not be limited by unnecessary restrictions.

> Colin's lung cancer had advanced rapidly, and despite the sterling efforts of his family and friends, he had to be admitted to hospital where he died within days. John paid many home visits to Colin, and then again to see the family after he had died. During his most recent visit John got a very strong sense from the family that they wanted assurance that they had done their best for Colin. Towards the end of the visit, John said: *'From a professional point of view, can I just say what a privilege it has been to work with you all. Not many families could have coped as well as you all have.'* There was a palpable feeling of relief that ran through the family.

Spontaneity

Spontaneity is using the right words at the right time. The words that a family doctor actually uses during a consultation are a mixture of memories and innovations. With age and experience there will tend to be more words used because of memories than because of innovations.

A family doctor needs some way of benchmarking to make sure that the words she has used are indeed the right words at the right time. Ways of doing this are suggested in Chapter 7 on training, involving reflection on consultations and the use of group work. When considering methods for improvement, the following pitfalls should be attended to.

- Words that are arrived at through innovation may be superficially attractive because of their novelty value. However, on balance they are less likely to be effective, since a family doctor usually commits a word or phrase to memory because it has previously been effective – it has a track record which the innovative word or phrase cannot (by definition) match. All clichés were at one time *bons mots*.
- It is a rare family doctor who will systematically assess the effect of previously used scripts. Feedback is based on intuition and general feelings about a

particular patient. Perhaps the family doctor's patient is just being nice to her by appearing to accept what she has said.

- Talk to your peers about which words to use. Each family doctor has only one lifetime of personal experience on which to draw. Not all consultation techniques work for all family doctors or indeed for all patients, but it makes sense for the family doctor to learn from the successes and failures of others when planning her own performance.
- What is said to a patient should be consistent with best medical communication practice. There may be applicable information of which the family doctor is unaware. A mistake is less likely to occur if more brains are brought to bear on the situation.
- What is said to a patient should be broadly consistent with what other family doctors are saying to patients. This does not mean that your performance should be invariably dreadful or 'dumbed down', but rather that it is important to ensure that patients are not receiving entirely conflicting information from different professional medical sources.

Realising that the start of a consultation is critical, John tried several different verbal openings to see which of them worked best. First up was *'How do you do?'*. This invariably produced the response *'Very well, thank you'*, after which the patient would go on to make it clear that they were far from being 'very well'. Next he tried *'What appears to be the problem?'*, but then he decided that this sounded rather patronising. Following an eavesdropping trip to the local town centre, he tried *'What's up now then?'* in a loud voice, but family doctors are not supposed to speak like that at all. He finally concluded that, after an initial 'hello' and possibly a brief prompt such as *'Well, now'* or *'What are we doing today?'*, his best strategy was to sit down, look at his patient, and wait.

Voice work

Family doctors spend a lot of their working time talking, but few give any thought to their voice and its improvement. The content of what is to be said was discussed earlier. However, the voice itself is also a crucial tool in communication. A family doctor's voice has to be 'heard' – in all senses of the word.

Consideration should be given to voice use and production. Using the voice properly means that what is said is more likely to be accurately received, and also avoids problems with voice strain. Most people are alarmed when they hear their voice on a tape recording. It is often not at all as they imagine it to be. One reason for this is that the sound heard by the outside listener is not the same as the sound heard by the speaker. Quirks of acoustics and distortions caused by sinuses and other resonant body cavities see to that. However, the other reason why the recorded voice sounds odd is because most speakers concentrate on what they are saying rather than listening for the sound that they produce.[18]

People typically try to use their voice for more than just the transmission of words. The words are important, of course, but then so too are the pauses and gaps between the words. Measured speech is associated with authority and confidence,[16] and also gives the speaker extra fractions of a second in which to choose the words more carefully and finish off the sentences.

People also try in their speech to convey emotion and emphasis through their narrative. This *signalling* – 'it ain't what you say, it's the way that you say it' – adds further meaning to the words that are used, and also makes the talk more interesting and therefore more memorable.

Relaxation

Being relaxed makes people feel and sound more authoritative and confident. A family doctor conducting a surgery is not quite as 'on display' as an actor on stage, but nevertheless there will be times when anxiety creeps into the proceedings. There may be an unaccustomed clinical situation, or the need to discuss some bad news, or there may just be an awkward patient to deal with. These are all situations where a family doctor will want to feel and appear to be in control.

Relaxation is cumulative. A spell of being relaxed has an effect on anxiety levels that lasts beyond the duration of the relaxation. This is why relaxation audiotapes and yoga work – a person does not have to be listening to the tape or sitting in the 'lotus position' all the time in order to get the benefit. On the other hand, spending more time relaxing, and particularly increasing the frequency of being relaxed, contributes to reducing background levels of anxiety. Regular relaxation makes for a more relaxed person.

The delivery of speech is all about articulation and the control of breathing. Breath control is not just about being able to speak loudly. It is also concerned with having enough breath and enough control to support the voice. When speaking to just one person in a confined space it is not usually necessary to speak loudly. However, it is important to be able to speak articulately and without breathiness, which requires just as much control as if one is trying to fill a large auditorium.

Most people do not use their voices to full effect because they are not able to access the depths and resonances by using the whole potential voice-production apparatus in their body. In particular, breath is commonly controlled by just the upper thorax, and only the throat is used to deliver the sound. More richness and variety of tone is produced if the lower thorax and particularly the diaphragm are used more. In the acting trade this is called *centring* the voice.

Some exercises to help with breath control and relaxation can be found in Chapter 7.

Summary

People have preconceptions and preferences concerning the kind of things they want or expect to hear. Words that do not accord with those preferences are unlikely to be fully understood, so finding out what the patient's preferences are is of some importance for a family doctor in consultation. In most (but not all) situations, patients prefer to be talked to in their own language and not in jargon or acronyms. Well-established verbal techniques exist to make communication more effective. The family doctor should try to make her consultations creative – that is, situations where patient and doctor are responding to each other and generating more than the sum of the parts. Spontaneity is using the right words at the right time – a mixture of innovation and memory. A family doctor's voice is an important consultation tool, so look after it.

References

1. Walter J and Bayat A (2003) Neurolinguistic programming: verbal communication. *BMJ Careers.* **15 March:** s83.
2. McKie R (2001) Whisper it quietly, but the power of language may be all in the genes. *Observer.* **7 October:** 14.
3. Silverman J, Kurtz S and Draper J (2004) *Skills for Communicating with Patients* (2e). Radcliffe Publishing, Oxford.
4. Pendleton D, Schofield T, Tate P *et al.* (1984) *The Consultation.* Oxford University Press, Oxford.
5. Helman CG (1994) *Culture, Health and Illness.* Butterworth Heinemann, Oxford.
6. Kindelan K and Kent G (1986) Patients' preferences for information. *J R Coll Gen Pract.* **36:** 461–3.
7. Baines E (2003) GPs advised to focus on forgetful patients. *Gen Practitioner.* **12 May:** 17.
8. Ley P (1977) Psychological studies of doctor–patient communication. In: S Rachman (ed.) *Contributions to Medical Psychology. Volume 1.* Pergamon Press, Oxford.
9. King A (2004) Hearing and the elderly: a simple cure. *Geriatr Med.* **34:** 9–15.
10. McCullough S (1989) Learning to talk. *GMC News Rev.* **September:** v–vi.
11. Fowler HW and Fowler FG (1964) *The Concise Oxford Dictionary.* Oxford University Press, Oxford.
12. Ogden J, Branson R, Bryett A *et al.* (2003) What's in a name? An experimental study of patients' views of the impact and function of a diagnosis. *Fam Pract.* **20:** 248–53.
13. Frazer J (1993) *The Golden Bough.* Wordsworth Editions, Ware.
14. Skelton JR, Wearn AM and Hobbs FDR (2002) 'I' and 'we': a concordancing analysis of how doctors and patients use first-person pronouns in primary care consultations. *Fam Pract.* **19:** 484–8.
15. Dobson R (2002) Sharing of uncertainty can unnerve patients. *BMJ.* **325:** 1319.
16. Dobson R (2002) Doctors fail to see the joke. *BMJ.* **325:** 561.
17. Johnstone K (1981) *Impro.* Methuen, London.
18. Berry C (1994) *Your Voice and How to Use It.* Virgin, London.

Chapter 7

Training for BARD

If a consultation technique cannot be learned and used by real family doctors in the real world, then it is a failure and not fit for its purpose. Most family doctors are constrained by the extreme pressure on their time and intellectual energy. Any training to develop a new technique or set of techniques must be achievable during everything else that is going on, and it should preferably show results straight away.

This chapter therefore works from the premise that the best training involves things that can be done alone, or with minimal outside involvement. The BARD training exercises suggested in this chapter can certainly be done in a group setting, but most of them can also be done by oneself.

A suitable group

If there is a group available, then by all means use it. A small group can achieve things that other learning formats cannot,[1] but not all family doctors have a suitable small group which they can utilise in this way. Family doctors in training will usually have a local group of peers, who offer an obvious source of a group. Newly qualified family doctors often get together for mutual support in the early years, and this also provides an ideal group opportunity.

Older family doctors may not have such a natural group to call upon. In addition, group work has to follow group aims, and each group member will certainly have their own agenda concerning what they want to achieve, which may be at variance with the agendas of the rest of the group. Indeed, older practitioners will often have a more clear and specific view of what they want to achieve from an educational event, and be less tolerant if their wishes are not fulfilled. Some family doctor trainers' groups offer appropriate support to experienced practitioners, but they will of necessity have an agenda that is rather different from the educational needs of participants.

Some of the issues that might be discussed are particularly sensitive, such as those which involve the competence of the participants, and especially where the personality and/or role of the family doctor is being discussed. If these areas can be discussed in a group setting, the potential advantages are considerable. However, it is a brave family doctor who will offer herself up to this kind of scrutiny. Some things are best reflected on alone, or else in a group that has a proven track record of sympathetic support.

Disclaimer

The exercises contained in this chapter are derived partly from training methods used by actors, and partly from established techniques used to train family doctor learners. They concentrate on some of the issues raised by the rest of the book, and are not intended to represent a comprehensive programme of consultation skills training.

Books written by actors for actors are fascinating, yet they look and feel rather unscientific. There is not a research base to support most of the theories. Much of the literature is written by famous actors rather than by teachers. There is a heavy dependence on the plays with which those actors have worked. The issues dealt with tend to be to do with interpersonal relationships and hidden motivations. There is of course a jargon to be learned, and comparisons, similes, analogies and anecdotes abound.

Chapter 2: role

The chapter on role set out an adapted version of the seven questions that Stanislavsky invited his acting students to address when developing a role for a theatrical performance.

Question 1   Who am I? What are my principles?

Aim:

To encourage the family doctor to think about what kind of family doctor she wants to be.

Method:

Reflect on the principles that guide your professional life.

In 2002, a theme issue of the *British Medical Journal* entitled 'What's a good doctor, and how can you make one?' attracted 102 responses from 24 countries, mostly from doctors themselves. Here is a selection of characteristics drawn from that source, to get the reflective ball rolling.[2-4]

A family doctor should be:

Respectful	Courteous
Unbiased	Able to work co-operatively in a team
Proactive	Conscientious/persistent
Authoritative	Accommodating
Attentive to patient needs	Self-analytical
Balanced	Brave
Caring	Competent
Compassionate	Confident
Creative	Decisive
Ethical	Able to show empathy
Energetic	Friendly
Faithful	Flexible
Gracious	Humorous
Humble	Intellectual
Informative	Wise in judgement

Kind	Loyal
Mature	Modest
Noble	Nurturing
Open-minded	Optimistic
Passionate	Patient
Positive	Realistic
Responsible	Sensitive
Selfless	Spiritual
Trustworthy	Thorough
Vigilant	Warm
Zestful	Up to date
Human	Responsive

Format:

1. Can be done alone, in which case the answers should be written down – they can then be referred to and amended later. Allow 30 minutes to do it properly.
2. Can also be done in a small group, but the group must be composed of trustworthy people who know you. A consensus view may emerge, which is right and proper. However, be sure that there is at least one respect in which your private views differ from the consensus views – take a stand for your individuality. Allow 20 minutes for general discussion, and a further 10 minutes per group member for the expression of individual opinions. Make sure that every group member (with their permission) is discussed during the same session.

A less personalised review of role might be addressed through a group discussion about more general issues, such as the collective ramifications of role. Examples of discussion topics might include the following.

- Should a family doctor always appear confident?
- Should a family doctor display emotion?
- What part should a family doctor play in local politics and the local community?
- What is meant by 'professionalism'?

Question 2   What has happened in my life to develop my principles?

Aims:

1. To consider the key life experiences that have resulted in current professional principles.
2. To consider how others (co-workers, patients) may have had different life experiences, resulting in their having different principles and priorities.

Method:

Reflect on significant life events and consider how they might have affected current principles. For example:

- family background

- educational experience
- personal/family illness or other mishap
- heroes
- religious or political beliefs
- lifestyle.

In addition, consider the following questions.

- If your patients were asked about your way of life, upbringing and education for your job as a family doctor, what do you think they would say?
- How does this match up to reality?

Format:

This is the same as for question 1. If it is done alone, allow up to 30 minutes, and write down the results. If it is done in a group, allow 20 minutes for general discussion, and then 10 minutes for each participant to relate their personal experiences, or one particularly significant experience.

Question 3   What order of priority do I give to my principles?

Aims:

1. To consider how you might respond if two or more professional principles were in conflict.
2. To consider what (if any) circumstances might cause the order of priorities to alter.

Methods:

1. Reflect on the list of principles discussed in question 1, and place them in rank order of importance.
2. Consider some problem professional scenarios and reflect on whether this rank order still applies. Examples might include the following:
   - using possibly fatal doses of opiates in a terminally ill patient
   - dealing with an under-performing colleague
   - addressing the contraceptive needs of a mentally disabled and vulnerable patient.

Format:

This exercise lends itself to personal reflection. Any group work should be preceded by the members making a personal prioritised list of their principles. These can then be discussed both generally and individually. The application of principles to the problem scenarios could certainly lead to lively group involvement. However, people who recognise that they have deeply held spiritual or political beliefs may find such discussions in a group setting a little disturbing.

Question 4   What are my inner characteristics?

Aims:

1. To consider what your personal emotional and thinking preferences are – that is, in what areas you are most comfortable – and to reflect on how this might affect your professional work.
2. To consider the implications of colleagues and patients who may have different preferences.

Method:

One instrument for identifying thinking preferences, namely the Myers–Briggs Type Indicator (MBTI), was discussed in Chapter 2 on role. Formal testing can certainly be done, but a strong indication of the outcome can be obtained by reflecting on the four pairs of characteristics used to express the results of testing. Such reflection requires a certain degree of personal honesty – there is nothing to be gained by either pomposity or false modesty. This part of the exercise should be done alone. Clubs and websites are available for members of different groups. For instance, http:/fuzzy.snakeden.org/intj/ has some very supportive and encouraging things to say about the INTJ type.

A group whose members have all been involved in a method of type testing will almost certainly welcome discussion of the method, results and implications for professional practice. It must be regularly emphasised that tools such as the MBTI indicate preferences and do not suggest that people are unable to behave or think in any other way.

Question 5   What do my patients and work colleagues think of me?

Aim:

To assess how near a family doctor is to fulfilling her professional principles.

Method:

Reflect on what you would say in a job interview situation if you were asked the following question: 'If we asked your colleagues and patients about you as a family doctor, what do you think they would say?'. How does this compare with the list of principles that you have identified for your professional role?

Consider the list of stakeholders offered in Chapter 4 (on aims). Look again at the list of desirable characteristics for a family doctor (Question 1). What sort of list of priorities do you think each of the stakeholders would draw up? How does it compare with your own list of priorities?

Format:

Both of these exercises may be done alone. When formulating an opinion, evidence should be used – a single lapse does not mean that everything is awful.

With one or two other people, you could role play the interview, with or without an observer. Considering the priorities of other stakeholders is something that would lend itself to group discussion after some preparatory work by the participants.

Question 6   Where am I?

Aim:

To consider how circumstances affect which aspects of the family doctor's chosen role are portrayed.

Method:

Reflect on how time affects the aspects of the role portrayed. This would include the following:

- the family doctor's age and experience
- how you did things when you were younger
- the age of the patient cohort that you usually see, the kind of problems that they have, and how long you have been seeing them for
- what the future is likely to bring.

Reflect on how place affects the aspects of the role portrayed. This would include the following:

- the social structure of the patient cohort
- the work and educational experience of the patient cohort
- the use of private medical services
- what the future is likely to bring.

Reflect on how context affects the aspects of the role portrayed. This would include the following:

- the age/sex composition of the rest of the workforce
- the weaknesses and strengths of the present organisation
- current political constraints on practice
- what the future is likely to bring.

Format:

This exercise can be done individually or as a group. Many of the issues will be specific to the family practice in which you are working, so a group consisting of fellow workers would probably be most productive. On the other hand, the internal politics might get in the way of free discussion.

Question 7   What long-term effects do I want?

Planning

Aims:

1. To consider what sort of reputation you have with your patients, how that reputation came about, and whether it is the reputation that you want.
2. To consider where you want to be professionally in the future.

Method:

Reflect on the following issues.

- Which parts of your professional and personal life do you wish to continue as now? (education, patient mix, organisation, work/life balance, etc.)
- Why have your regular patients become regulars?
- Which parts of your professional and personal life would you like to change?
- How will you bring about those changes, and when?
- What internal and external factors may affect any changes?
- Describe your working day one year, five years and 10 years from now.

Format:

This exercise is best done alone. It is a good idea to write down the results of the reflection. If it can be arranged, write down your thoughts in the form of a letter to yourself, and then ask someone to give it back to you in a year's time. The exercise can be done remarkably quickly – within 10 to 20 minutes – but it will feel as if it takes rather longer.

Effect of patients

Aim:

To recognise and consider how you respond, both personally and professionally, to patient consulting behaviour.

Method:

Think back to two recent consultations, one with a patient whom you know well, and another with a patient you are meeting for the first time.

- Did you feel satisfied at the end of these consultations?
- What did the patients say or do that made you feel more satisfied?
- What did the patients say or do that made you feel less satisfied?
- Are you looking forward to consulting with these particular patients again?
- At the end of the consultations, did you feel ready to face:
  - the next patient
  - the rest of the day
  - the rest of your working career?

Format:

If this exercise is done alone, a recording will help to emphasise the behavioural specifics of what happened. Allow 10 minutes for reflection.

A group is better for this exercise. Triumphs are sweeter, and disasters are diluted and sympathised with. There is necessary discussion about background and your feelings. Allow 15 minutes for each case that is discussed.

Chapter 3: behaviour

Status

Aims:

1. To be able to project high and low status in a consultation.
2. To be sensitive to the status implications of family doctor and patient behaviour during a consultation.

Methods:

1. Reflect on a recent consultation.
   - Did you feel of high or low status during the consultation?
   - What did you do to project high status?
   - What did you do to project low status?
   - Was your status projection appropriate?
   - What was the effect of the status that you projected?
   (*See* Chapter 3 for examples of high- and low-status projection behaviours.)
2. During a communication situation, choose one or more of the characteristic traits of high status, and try them out.
   - How did you feel? Better than normal? Worse than normal? The same as normal? (You may be naturally dominant.)
   - How did the people with whom you were communicating behave? Did they appear content or uneasy? Did they reflexly display any passive traits?
3. In a communication situation, try to move gradually from high to low status (or from low to high status).
   - How did you feel? Was this an artificial or a natural-feeling communication?
   - What behaviour was used by the person(s) with whom you were communicating?
4. Choose a communication situation involving people whose self-esteem is secure and who can handle a joke. Play high status outrageously, and you will look like a complete idiot. Then try playing over-the-top low status, and be surprised at how much control you have.

Format:

This exercise can be done alone, by reflecting on the status behaviour used in a recent consultation.

It is also possible to do this exercise while consulting. Since you are already projecting status when consulting, it is acceptable to deliberately try out some high- or low-status behaviours and observe the effects on both you and your patients.

Ideas concerning status can also be discussed in a group situation. In addition, there will already be some jockeying for status within the group, so you might as well join in the game.

In a small social gathering, playing very high or very low status is usually good for a laugh.

A large social gathering is not the most obvious resource for professional training, you might think, but in fact it is ideal for trying out some of the facial expression and eye contact tricks associated with high status.

Video recording

Video is clearly the best way yet devised for seeing what really happens during a consultation. There can be no hiding – whatever you think you did, the recording shows what you actually did.

However, video recording does have limitations. The presence of the video camera may well alter doctor and patient behaviour, and there is evidence that patients who agree to be videoed differ from those who do not.[5]

The playing back and analysis of videoed consultations always takes a lot more time than you think it will.

Aim:

To focus on specific behaviour used during a consultation.

Method:

Two techniques worth trying are either to keep stopping the video to look at particular points, or to discuss the video in its entirety.

Interrupting the video
- What status are you playing, and why?
- Comment on your own and your patient's body language.
- Does your demeanour appear as intended?
- Have you used that behaviour before? If so, what was the context and what was the effect?
- What behavioural options did you have at this point?

Discussing the video in its entirety
- Did your behaviour portray a consistent overall image, or was there scope for confusion?
- If there were inconsistencies, what was the reason for them? Were they intentional? Were they intuitive? Were they mistakes?
- Was the overall image portrayed the one that was intended?
- Was your personal image elevated or lowered?
- Was the image of the profession elevated or lowered?

Format:

Video work can be done alone. It can still be embarrassing, but is less stressful than when viewed in a group. It is difficult to be completely objective about your own behaviour. Allow at least twice as long as the consultation.

Group video work can involve two or more people. The opportunity for both critical examination and support is greater – most family doctors are more critical of their own performance than they would be about someone else's. It may be tempting to 'tough it out' to save embarrassment, rather than to remain objective. You should always use Pendleton's rules[6] (*see* Appendix 7.5) or another feedback system. Allow at least four times as long as the duration of the consultation, as there will be explaining to do as well as analysis of the video.

Role play

Role play is an excellent way of practising communication and behavioural skills in a way that can't possibly harm patients.

Role play is easy, cheap and always available. In fact it can be inserted into other learning situations. Two specific educational benefits are that a family doctor can be asked to play the patient role (which in itself can be a significant educational experience), and the same 'scenes' can be run repeatedly to reinforce the learning. On the other hand, participants in role play may have trouble 'losing' their medical perspective when looking at communication issues. Observers may make suggestions that they have found work for them, but with which the role player does not feel comfortable.

Aims:

1. To focus on specific behaviour that might be used in consultations.
2. To encourage the consideration and practice of behavioural options.
3. To experience what it is like to be on the receiving end of a consultation.

Method:

A minimum of two people is needed, and some preparation is necessary. The participants will present or have written up brief scenarios of roles to play. If this is reinforced with a video recording, so much the better. An alternative is to use some of the published scenarios, and for this you could do a lot worse than refer to *The Consultation Toolkit.*[7]

Ways to use role play include the following.[8]

- *Mini role play*, to look at specific phases in a consultation – for instance, to find out if a patient with a headache is worried that he might have a brain tumour.
- *Prepared role play*, to look at a larger topic – for instance, disclosing to a patient and their family a diagnosis of dementia.
- *Reverse role play*, where a participant brings a problem case and it is played out with the participant taking the role of the 'patient' – for instance, a request for a PSA test in an asymptomatic man.
- *'Good doctor, bad doctor'*, where a deliberately bad performance is offered – good for light relief, and to convince participants that however badly they think things went, they could always have been worse.

Format:

This exercise cannot be done alone. If a group is available, it should be divided into twos (patient and family doctor) and threes (patient, family doctor and observer).

Written notes can be useful. All of the participants must be prepared to role play. Knowing the other participants is less important than for other group activities, as you will intuitively modify your behaviour towards what you are comfortable displaying to the specific audience.

Each scenario will take about twice as long in a role-play situation as it would in a real consultation. At least as much time again should be allowed for discussion. Each member of the group of two or three should have a chance to play patient, family doctor and (if present) observer.

The role play can be video recorded for later use.

Displaying emotion

According to the Stanislavsky school, the most realistic portrayal of an emotion occurs when the portrayer recalls from their memory an instance when they felt the emotion in a real situation, and then duplicates the behaviour which was used at that time.

Aims:

1. To become more aware of the emotions that are generated in a consultation – for both the family doctor and the patient.
2. To be able to portray an emotion in a consultation when the situation requires it.

Method:

Reflect on two recent consultations, one where you felt a strong emotion and one where your patient displayed a strong emotion.

- How would you describe the emotion that you felt?
- Did you display the emotion outwardly? How? Why?
- Did your display of emotion alter the consultation? If so, in what respect?
- Did your behaviour change after your patient displayed their strong emotion?

Reflection/discussion topics
- Is it ever appropriate for a family doctor to display powerful emotion when consulting?
- Have you ever been angry, elated or distressed during a consultation? What did you do and say – that is, what behaviour did you use?

Format:

Much of this can be done alone. Indeed it might be more comfortable to do the exercises alone. A video of a real case (if available) may help.

If any of these exercises are done in a group, that group must be characterised by mutual trust. Since the way in which emotion is portrayed is very personal, comments are appropriate but advice about how to 'do it better' is not.

Chapter 4: aims

Aim setting

Aims:

1. To be as focused as possible about what you are trying to achieve in a consultation.
2. To appreciate the wide range of legitimate aims that are possible when consulting.

Method:

Reflect on a recent consultation. Write down what your aims were for that consultation – try and find one for each category of aim. Include aims from the start of the consultation, those that emerged as the consultation proceeded, and any that were left over for the next consultation(s). The categories are as follows:

- clinical aims
- professional aims
- social aims
- organisational aims
- personal aims.

(*See* Chapter 4 on aims for a fuller discussion of these categories.)

Format:

First-level completion is the ability to articulate and write down your aims for a consultation after it has happened.

Second-level completion is the ability to explain to a group what you were doing and why you were doing it. A video is useful here.

Obstacles

Aim:

To be aware of the options available for achieving an aim.

Method:

Reflect on a consultation in which things did not go according to plan.

- What were the aim(s) that were not achieved?
- How important or significant was it that particular aim(s) should be achieved? Does it matter?
- Were there any resource factors that hindered achievement of the aim(s)?
- Were there any patient characteristics that hindered achievement of the aim(s)? For example:
  - locus of control (*see* Chapter 6 on dialogue)
  - expectations
  - personality/attitudes
  - type of problem?
- Were there any family doctor factors that hindered achievement of the aim(s)? For example:
  - knowledge
  - skills
  - attitudes
  - mood at the time?

Format:

It is probably best to do this exercise alone. Only you will really know what was in your mind at the time of the consultation – but be honest with yourself.

Members of a group may be able to offer third-party insight into events, and possibly suggest alternative behaviours. A description of the consultation is often enough – a video is the icing on the cake.

Long-term aims

Aim:

To be aware that each consultation has implications for future consultations. A reputation is being formed.

Method:

Reflect on two recent consultations, one with a patient you know well and one with a patient you are meeting for the first time. For each of them, consider the following.

- What were the aim(s) for the consultation which might have long-term implications?
- Did this consultation show you in the intended light?
- What happened in the consultation to promote these long-term aim(s)?

- What happened in the consultation which might have hindered the achievement of these aims?
- Will you behave in the same manner when you see this patient again, or will you try to behave differently?

Format:

Do this exercise alone.

If a group is available, the exercise may prompt discussion of whether there is or should be a consensus about the role of the family doctor, and how individual family doctors seek to promote that role.

Conflicting aims

Aim:

To be aware that patients also have aims for a consultation, which may well conflict with your own aims.

Method:

This exercise should be done in pairs. The participants play the roles of 'family doctor' or 'patient'. Each is given an aim for the consultation, and in addition the 'patient' has a very brief clinical scenario. The participants do not know each other's aim.

The pair role play, and time is called when one participant knows what the other's aim is.

Suggested family doctor aims

- I want to make myself look clever.
- I want to get on to the next patient.
- This consultation is being videoed for the MRCGP exam.
- I do not want to get involved long term with this patient.
- I want to make myself look warm, compassionate and caring.
- I know that this patient has been abrasive towards the reception staff. I want to make it clear that I know there has been a problem and that I am supporting my staff.

Suggested patient aims

- I have had this bad back for years, and I want some tests to find out what it is.
- I have had a bad sore throat which is now getting better, but I want the doctor to know that I would have come to see about it last week if the triage nurse had not put me off.
- I know I have prostate trouble, and I want to be referred to a specialist.
- I have a troublesome cough, and I know that if I am nice enough to the doctor then he or she will take pity on me and cure it.

Continued

> • I have an itchy rash on my arm. I have read in the *Daily Mail* that the only way to get a half decent service from a nationalised health service is either to complain, or to look as if I am going to complain.

Format:

This exercise needs two people. If there are more, they can be divided into twos, with any that are left over functioning as observers or note keepers.

In a group, all of the pairs can be role playing at the same time. The scenarios can be swapped and changed.

Allow 10 minutes for each role play, and allow a further 10 minutes for discussion of the behaviour and words used to achieve the aim.

Consider the following questions.

• Did the behaviour that you used communicate the chosen image effectively? If not, why not?
• What behaviour would be appropriate for:
  – the sympathetic family doctor
  – the patient's friend
  – the distinguished family doctor
  – the efficient family doctor
  – the up-to-date family doctor?
• What, from your personal perspective, are the advantages and disadvantages of each approach?

Chapter 5: room

Aim:

To be aware of the effects of the physical environment on the conduct of consultations.

Method:

By referring to your own experience, consider each of the following issues.

• What are the advantages and disadvantages, from the perspective of all of the stakeholders, of a family doctor consulting with patients:
  – at the surgery
  – during a routine home visit
  – during an emergency home visit
  – in a public place?
  (*See* Chapter 4 on aims for examples of stakeholders.)
• Consider the last time you consulted with a patient in a public place. What feelings did you have before, during and after the consultation? Comparing this consultation with a typical consultation in the surgery, did you have to adapt your clinical or communication behaviour? If so, in what respects?
• Where do you prefer to consult with patients? Why? Where do you think your patients would prefer to consult?
• Have you made any changes to your consulting room to make it more:
  – family doctor-friendly

– patient-friendly?

What did you do? Was there an event that prompted the change? Did the change have the desired effect, and how do you know that it did?

- Take a 'patient journey' through your surgery, starting outside, moving into the waiting room, and then into the consulting room to sit in the patient's chair. What do you notice? What feelings are generated?
- Reflect on an important visit you have made – for example, to a courtroom, solicitor, accountant or your own family doctor. What physical features did you notice? What feelings did the environment generate in you? How did you feel compared with your feelings when consulting? Did you feel confident? Did you feel in control? Were you thinking clearly?
- Reflect on a recent consultation. What equipment did you use during the consultation? Did you make any movements around the room? Reflect both on the behaviour and on your thoughts at the time. Was your physical movement related to one or more consultation aims?

Format:

These exercises can be done as effectively alone as in a group. Some general issues concerning surgery design can readily be shared with others in a group. You might even be invited to look around another family doctor's surgery, which is always a fascinating experience.

Chapter 6: dialogue

Creativity

Being verbally creative is a way of making a consultation unique and per-sonalised. If they allow themselves to be, people are more creative than you might expect. Listen to children explaining to their parents when they have been naughty. Listen to adults describing a situation in such a way that they could not possibly be in the wrong. Listen to politicians and lawyers nearly all the time.

Imagine that you are walking in the park with a dog.

- What colour is the dog?
- How big is he?
- Does he have a collar?
- Is he on a lead?
- How long is the lead?
- Call the dog by his name.
- What has he found in the grass?
- What does it smell like?
- Is the dog trying to lick it?
- The dog picks it up to take it home. What do you do?

If you found that exercise at all difficult, it was probably because you were trying to choose the most interesting or novel answer to each question. You probably had a lot of ideas, yet deliberately rejected most of them. The ideas are not the problem – it's what you choose to do with them. Try again, but this time use the very first idea, however boring or bizarre, that pops into your head. Now you are being creative.

Aim:

To encourage the use of, and confidence in, creative thinking in a consultation.

Methods:

These exercises are adapted from improvisation techniques used to train actors. Two or three people are given a brief scenario to act out. If the scenario is a medical one, then it must be one which none of the participants has dealt with. There are a number of suitable examples in *The Consultation Toolkit.*[7] However, to make sure that entrenched habits do not intrude, it may be better to use non-medical scenarios.

- *Two places.* Invite the participants to interact on the basis that there is disagreement about where they are. For instance, one believes that they are waiting at a bus-stop while the other believes that they are in his sitting room.
- *Experts.* The participants are an interviewer and an interviewee. The latter has to pretend to be a convincing expert on whatever topic the interviewer chooses. The expert is introduced with an introductory sentence, preferably one that the interviewer starts without knowing how it is going to end. *'Good evening. We are fortunate to have Professor Trout in the studio with us, who has just returned from Africa where he has been teaching hippopotamuses to. . . .'* Insert anything here – *'do handstands'*, *'yodel'*, *'knit'*.
- *Word at a time.* In rotation, each of the participants offers a single word in a narrative, the only rule being that everyone should try not to give the last word of a sentence.
- *Verbal chase.* This is a good game, especially if you have access to a resource who is used to teaching improvisation, such as an actor or someone from the local drama school. It is rather like the game with the dog in the park (see above). The questions and answers must be delivered rapidly (*see* example in Appendix 7.1).

And a couple of sneaky ones.

- *Random answers.* Set up a clinical scenario, and tell the 'patient' (without telling the 'family doctor') to answer in the affirmative any question that ends in a vowel, and negatively any question that ends in a consonant (*see* Appendix 7.2 for an example).
- *Yes, but.* This is a scenario where a family doctor is offering advice. To each question the 'patient' should agree and then offer a reservation (*see* Appendix 7.3 for an example).

Format:

This exercise cannot be done alone. At least two people are needed, and any others can act as observers. Each scenario is brief, and will be over in a matter of seconds.

Each group member should have the opportunity to participate, and then to reciprocate with the same or another partner. Involvement is the best way of learning, but the shy must be given the option of just observing.

Spontaneity

Aim:

To be able to choose the right words during a consultation.

Method:

'Acceptors' are people who will make the best of what is given to them, and respond appreciatively. They tend to answer questions with a 'yes', and they are rewarded with novelty and excitement. Accepting an offer creates warmth within the relationship. 'Blockers' instinctively answer questions in the negative. They are scared of anything new and different, and their punishment is a boring life, and being boring to others.

Work through a role play of a potentially difficult consultation. The family doctor should first play an 'acceptor' and then play a 'blocker'. Examples are given in Appendix 7.4. The words and behaviour that are used, and the feelings that are generated, are all relevant.

Format:

This exercise needs at least two people, but an audience is also permissible.

The best clinical scenarios to use are those that one of the participants experienced for real and had problems with.

Voice work

Voice exercises

These exercises have been designed to train actors.[9] Even if you feel completely happy with your vocal delivery, the exercises may help you to realise that there may be even more in the tank. Most of them can be done either lying down or standing. If they are done lying down they focus more on relaxation. If they are done standing they give a better preparation for the situations in which they are going to be of use.

Posture

Chest out, shoulders back, buttocks tucked in. This should not feel tense, and if it does you are trying too hard. If you have difficulty with this, try the exercises that physiotherapists use to help people who have repeated episodes of back pain.

Neck exercises

Let your head drop first forward, then backwards, and then to either side. Try and keep your shoulders completely relaxed. As you move your head upright again, try and be aware of the tension in the muscles that you are using.

With your head upright, push it backwards and feel the tension in the nuchals. Then push your chin down a bit and feel the different tension that is produced.

Roll your head around without twisting your neck. Roll it a long way at first. Then stop and try again, but this time moving it only fractionally. Stay aware of the tension that is produced in your neck muscles.

Shoulder exercise

Lift your shoulders up about half an inch, and then let them drop again. Make sure that you don't stoop. Let your shoulders fall a little below where they started, and be aware of the feeling in the muscles.

First breathing exercise

Put your hands behind your head with your elbows abducted. Breathe in slowly through your nose and without moving your shoulders. Let the breath out with a sigh, and keep exhaling until all of the breath has gone. When you feel the need, inhale again and let the breath out in the same manner. Repeat this six times.

Second breathing exercise

Place your hands over your lower ribs. Keeping your neck and shoulders relaxed, breathe in by expanding the lower thoracic diameter – there should be a pressure from your hands. Be aware of the sensation in your lower intercostals. Exhale with a sigh. Repeat this three times. This exercise should be quite tiring if you are doing it properly.

Third breathing exercise

Put one hand on your lower ribs, and the other over your xiphisternum. As you inhale this time, feel your lower ribs moving, but at the same time get your diaphragm moving – this will involve some distension of the upper abdomen. Sigh the breath away, but centre the sigh on the upper abdomen. Do this again, but instead of an exhalation sigh, make an 'er' noise, then 'ay', then 'I'. And finally try a few words delivered from the diaphragm – a nursery rhyme will do.

A pre-delivery checklist[9]

- Is the posture correct?
- Are the neck and shoulders relaxed?
- Are the lower intercostals and diaphragm primed for action?

A delivery checklist

- Is the throat open?
- Is the sound centred?
- Is the chest contributing to the sound?

In addition to these basic breathing and relaxation exercises, other speech exercises have been devised to help with enunciation. If needed, they should be looked up in a suitable book – for instance, *Your Voice and How to Use It.*[9]

Tape recorder

These days, even cheap tape recorders are good enough to give an accurate idea of how your voice sounds to the outside world. Recordings can be made 'before and after' you have done the above exercises. Have they made a difference? Do you like the changes? Audio recording can also be used during actual consultations, subject to obtaining appropriate permission from the patients involved. This avoids the visual distraction of a videoed consultation, and allows you to concentrate solely on what is said and how it is said.

Audio recording is currently little used for training in the consultation. This is a pity. Visual images are so strong that the verbal communication which is going on can easily be lost. Some of the early analysis of real consultations was done using audio recordings,[10] and it is possible to glean nearly as much information from these as from the now conventional video recording.

Listening to an audio recording of your consultations can be done alone but, as with video analysis, is probably more useful if done with one or more others. The 'rules of engagement' should be those described by Pendleton *et al.*[6] for video analysis.

References

1. Lewis B (1996) Getting the best from group work. *Training Update.* **April:** 10–12.
2. Rizo CA, Jadad AR and Enkin M (2002) Doctors should be good companions for people (letter). *BMJ.* **325**: 711.
3. Parmar MS (2002) ABC of being a good doctor (letter). *BMJ.* **325**: 711.
4. Coulter A (2002) Patients' views of the good doctor. *BMJ.* **325**: 668–9.
5. Coleman T and Manku-Scott T (1998) Comparison of video-recorded consultations in which patient consent is withheld. *Br J Gen Pract.* **48**: 971–4.
6. Pendleton D, Schofield T, Tate P *et al.* (1984) *The Consultation: an approach to teaching and learning.* Oxford University Press, Oxford.
7. Druquer M and Hutchinson S (2000) *The Consultation Toolkit.* Reed Healthcare Publishing, Sutton.
8. Kurtz S, Silverman J and Draper J (2004) *Teaching and Learning Communication Skills in Medicine* (2e). Radcliffe Publishing, Oxford.
9. Berry C (1994) *Your Voice and How to Use It.* Virgin, London.
10. Byrne PS and Long BEL (1976) *Doctors Talking to Patients.* HMSO, London.
11. Johnstone K (1981) *Impro.* Methuen, London.

Verbal chase

An example from a real-life situation of actor training[11]

'Where are you?'
'Here.'
'You're not. Where are you?'
'In a box.'
'Who put you there?'
'Mummy.'
'She's not really your mummy. Who is she?'
'She's my aunt.'
'What's her secret plan?'
'To kill me.'
'With what?'
'A knife.'
'She sticks the knife where?'
'In . . . . in . . . . in my stomach.'
'She cuts it open and takes out a handful of papery . . .?'
'Boxes.'
'On the boxes is written . . .?'
'Help.'
'Who wrote it?'
'I did.'

Random answers

Another game to be played in pairs emphasises the potential creativity of a consultation conversation. The consultation is about a possible urinary tract infection in a young woman. The game is a device for making sure that neither participant knows what is going to happen next. The best improvisers are those who 'walk into a room backwards' – they know where they have come from but have no preconceptions about where they are going.[11] The 'doctor' must ask only questions that can be answered with a 'yes' or 'no' response. Without the 'doctor's' knowledge, the 'patient' is asked to answer in the affirmative if the doctor's question ends in a vowel, and negatively if it ends in a consonant. It is amazing how far you can get down the management track without the consultation seizing up.

Random answers

Patient:	'I think I've got a water infection.'
Family doctor:	'Is your water burning you?'
Patient:	'Yes, it is. It feels really hot.'
Family doctor:	'And are you going a lot?'
Patient:	'No, not really.'
Family doctor:	'What about in the night? Do you have to get up in the night to make water?'
Patient:	'Not at all. I'm quite all right with that.'
Family doctor:	'So it hurts when you pass water, but you are not going any more than usual?'
Patient:	'No, you don't seem to understand. I think I've got a water infection.'
Family doctor:	'OK. What about a discharge from your vagina?'
Patient:	'Oh yes. I've had one of those for two weeks.'
Family doctor:	'Now then, we may be on to something here. Is the discharge thick and creamy?'
Patient:	'No, it's not like that at all.'
Family doctor:	'It sounds like it's not something simple like thrush. I had better get a specimen off to the lab before deciding on the best treatment.'

Yes, but . . .

Family doctor:	'You told me last week that you gave up smoking after your heart attack, but then I saw you yesterday smoking in the street.'
Patient:	'Yes, but it was only one.'
Family doctor:	'Come off it – I can smell it on your clothes.'
Patient:	'Yes, but I took the wife out for a drink in a smoky pub yesterday.'
Family doctor:	'You know that it's dangerous for you to smoke, especially now that you have got heart trouble.'
Patient:	'Yes, but you told me that my heart had healed, and that if I take my cholesterol tablets it won't happen again.'
Family doctor:	'The only person you are harming is yourself.'
Patient:	'Yes, but a cig does calm my nerves, and being nervous leads to heart attacks.'
Family doctor:	'You know you are being silly, don't you?'
Patient:	'Yes, but I've always been silly, and it's a bit late to change now.'

Acceptors and blockers

This patient has recently been diagnosed as hypertensive and has been having trouble with the side-effects of treatment. He has now come to see his family doctor because he wants to be referred to a specialist.

Patient:	'I want to see a specialist about my blood pressure.'
Family doctor:	'I see. And why would that be, then?'
Patient:	'It's just that I know you are very busy and I thought a specialist might know more . . . have more experience . . . you know what I mean.'
Family doctor:	'Now look here, I am quite capable of treating a simple case of blood pressure, you know.'
Patient:	'I'm sorry. I really didn't mean to imply that you were no good. I really am very happy with what you have done. But high blood pressure is important, isn't it?'
Family doctor:	'You are right, blood pressure is very important. A pity you didn't think of that when you began to put on weight and gave up exercise.'
Patient:	'I think a patient has a right to see a specialist if he wants to.'
Family doctor:	'We can't go wasting taxpayers' money on sending you to hospital with something which can be dealt with quite adequately without.'
Patient:	'If I pay, can't I see a specialist?'
Family doctor:	'I suppose I can't stop you wasting your own money, if you must.'

Or, alternatively:

Patient:	'I want to see a specialist about my blood pressure.'
Family doctor:	'That sounds like a good idea. Was there anything in particular that you hoped the specialist would be able to help you with?'
Patient:	'You know I have been getting all these side-effects from the tablets. The thought of having to take them for the rest of my life really depresses me.'
Family doctor:	'Yes, I can see that it might. I'll do a letter for a really good chap at the General who will be sure to get you on the right lines. But it will take a bit of time to arrange, so what shall we do while we're waiting?'
Patient:	'How do you mean?'
Family doctor:	'Well, for instance, there might be ways other than tablets to get your blood pressure down. Is it worth a try?'

Pendleton's rules

Pendleton's rules are derived from the book *The Consultation: an approach to teaching and learning*,[6] and originally referred to the situation of giving feedback on video-recorded consultations. They can be summarised as follows.

- Briefly clarify and provide matters of fact.
- The doctor in question goes first.
- Give the good points first.
- Make recommendations, not criticisms.

Chapter 8

The ethics of BARD

BARD is different from other and established models of the family medicine consultation. It is not task based, it makes suggestions about the limits to which a family doctor can work, it emphasises that family doctors (and indeed other people) also have legitimate rights in their dealings with their patients, and it offers a means by which family doctors can more fully express their personality through their work. BARD is a more accurate reflection of how real family doctors conduct their consultations, and celebrates this reality rather than bemoaning the fact that what family doctors actually do falls short of what they should do.

Because the model is new and goes against the current trend, many will be concerned both about whether BARD can be done, and also about whether it should be done. Changes in consulting technique should rightly be resisted unless they are likely to bring about an improvement. In addition, consideration should be given to whether BARD breaches the ethical principles by which family doctors conduct their professional responsibilities.

Is BARD 'patient-centred'?

> Patient-centredness is at the heart of medicine. It is a core value of our discipline, recognised as the best way of helping an individual promote, preserve and restore their integrity of health. Patient-centredness is about giving the patient's viewpoints much more status in our hierarchy of clinical inputs . . .[1]

It would be hard to envisage a more fulsome endorsement of patient-centredness than the above quotation from an editorial in the *British Journal of General Practice*. It recognises that for many years a family doctor could fully expect her patients to do as they were told. If they did not comply with her orders, they had only themselves to blame for their illness. What is the point of consulting an expert if you do not then follow their advice? Such an attitude no longer makes sense (if it ever did). In the first place, the best medical outcomes are obtained only when patients are involved in making decisions about their care. This requires that the information needed to make such decisions is fully communicated. Only when ideas, concerns and expectations have been explored can a complete diagnosis of the problem be made. An autocratic family doctor is a medically deficient family doctor. Secondly, investing all of the authority in a family medicine consultation with the doctor is undemocratic, ignores the public service role that family doctors should play in society, and is incompatible with the rise of consumer power and the demand for increasing accountability from professional groups of all kinds. Doctor-centred medicine is ethically unsound.

BARD fully recognises the need for patient-centredness, but takes this a stage further. Much of the good that derives from a consultation in family practice comes from the quality of the relationship that the participants generate. Each has their own individual expertise to contribute, and true collaboration occurs when each point of view is assimilated. Being patient-centred is not the same as never offering a patient who needs it unqualified support and comfort. Being patient-centred is not the same as passing over to a patient all management decisions without making it clear that some options are medically better than others. Being patient-centred is not the same as never having a medical opinion – an expressed assessment, taking all of the factors into account, of what a family doctor believes is in the best interests of her patient. When family doctors and patients can interact at a personal level as well as at a professional and scientific one, the degree of understanding is maximised, as well as the potential benefits from the consultation. Family doctors should not be obliged to obey without question what their patients tell them any more than patients should be obliged to obey their family doctor. By accepting that the participants are human, a BARD consultation is one in which both participants can flourish.

What of the other stakeholders that BARD suggests have a legitimate interest in a consultation? Does this make the consultation less patient-centred? Accepting that other stakeholders exist does no more than reflect the reality of the circumstances under which family doctors work. Many family doctors would love a working life that did not include managers, healthcare payers, politicians and lawyers, and that allowed them to concentrate exclusively on the interests of the patient in front of them. However, this does not equate with the real world. The strength of BARD is that it recognises the different stakeholders so that the family doctor can adjust accordingly. Different stakeholders are playing out their own roles and pursuing their own agendas, and decisions can be made about how much notice is going to be taken of each group. By being much clearer about the things that might obstruct patient-centredness, the BARD family doctor is likely to be more rather than less patient-centred in her approach.

Who chooses a family doctor's role?

A defining feature of family doctors is that they aspire to address the primary care needs of their patients. The work they do is mainly demand led, and their purpose is to deal with any issue that a patient chooses to present to them. They are truly the servants of their patients. If this is the case, then patients and society should decide what a family doctor should do. However, BARD suggests that the work of a family doctor involves more than just attending to patient wants or needs, and that the family doctor should define for herself a role which has aspects that are separate from the services which she offers to her patients. Is this view justifiable?

In this book the chapters on role and behaviour argued that, despite attempts to offer a definition of a family doctor in terms of the jobs that she does, a good deal of the relationship between a family doctor and her patients is based on trust. It is not possible to draw up a contract with enough detail and flexibility to cover all of the nuances that a typical consultation in family practice contains. A job description is necessary because it provides the basis for regulation of the profession, and it gives an idea of what patients can reasonably expect from a consultation, but it does not sufficiently describe all that is going on. In addition, a job description tells the family doctor what to do, but does not tell her how to do it.

The role that a BARD family doctor chooses is her set of professional principles – the motivators that direct her work. Her principles will influence how she fulfils her job description. The social dimensions of the family doctor's role are those principles on which nearly all family doctors would agree. An individual BARD family doctor's chosen role will be consistent with these social dimensions of role, but with the added element of the personal principles which make her contribution to the care of her patients unique. The principles will be sincerely held (otherwise they would not be principles), and so will of necessity affect everything that she does in her professional duties.

Which aspects of role are on display?

BARD suggests that the principles that a family doctor employs in her professional role are a subset of the principles that she employs in her total existence – consistent with, but separate. Does this mean that patients are engaging with an incomplete personality, and that a family doctor always keeps some things secret from her patients? BARD also suggests that keeping a distance (however small) between her person and her professional role helps the family doctor to deal with criticism of her role without feeling that this is also an attack on her person. Is this fair on the patient who actually wants to attack the family doctor at a personal level?

The principles that a family doctor uses, and the priority that is given to those principles, are both situation-specific. The principles that are prominent in the family doctor's domestic life are not the same as the principles that are most prominent in her professional work. This is unexceptional – all people adjust their priorities according to circumstances, and it would be wrong to expect a family doctor to be any different in this respect.

As long as a family doctor behaves towards her patients in accordance with her professional role, critics have no legitimate avenues of attack other than to attack the role and/or the behaviour. Critics may make assumptions about the fundamental nature (the person) of their object of criticism, but these remain assumptions and essentially unprovable, as the only evidence they have is the observed behaviour. It is most unlikely that a family doctor would deliberately set out to injure a patient, so criticism of a family doctor's role is difficult to substantiate. If a patient has a bad outcome, then it is much more likely to be either the result of a mistake (the family doctor's behaviour was wrong), or bad luck. Mistakes can be analysed and learned from, whereas bad luck is just bad luck.

Trust is an inevitable component of the relationship between an expert and a non-expert, and it has personal as well as social components. Patients have trust in all family doctors, and in addition they have specific trust in the family doctors with whom they have dealings, trust which is experienced at a personal level. If this trust is thought to have been betrayed, then there will be social and personal dimensions to the sense of betrayal, and hence the motivation to launch an attack at a personal level. However, the non-expert may not be able to comprehend that the expert role is distinct from the person pursuing the role, so that criticisms concerning the relevant area of expertise are always objectively attacks on role or behaviour, whatever the intention of the attacker. Critics may direct their criticisms in a personal way, but it would be an unprofessional family doctor who was prepared to receive them in this form.

'No gain without pain'

It is difficult to challenge the morals of a family doctor who overworks. Generations of medical families have put up with a perpetually absent parent – behaviour which in most other jobs would be deemed a dereliction of parental duty – on the justification that the errant family doctor was off doing good things for her patients. Family practice offers plenty of good excuses not to be at home. Traditional models of the consultation suggest great rafts of tasks which should be done in a consultation, the family doctor's input becoming ever more intensive and painstaking. It would seem that, so far as a consultation in primary care is concerned, the more work that the family doctor puts in and the more personal pain she endures, the better the outcome will be for her patient.

The majority of family doctors believe that they are working hard already. In this they are no different from other people – being thought 'lazy' is pejorative in most cultures. On the other hand, the evidence of the prevalence of stress-related disorders would suggest that family doctors have a better case than many for considering themselves overworked. Inviting family doctors to work harder still is not sensible. Resources are not available to allow family doctors to perform longer and more intensive consultations while at the same time maintaining the accessibility that patients and governments seem to require. In any case, the way in which a family doctor uses her personality, and the quality of the relationships that develop with patients, are more important in determining consultation outcome than the energy expenditure and anguish experienced by the family doctor.[2]

BARD suggests that it is a reasonable and legitimate aim for every consultation that the family doctor takes steps to protect her own health. A mentally and/or physically ill family doctor will not only be suffering herself, but will also be delivering a sub-optimal service to her patients. Family doctors already use coping strategies, and it is likely that the ones who use their strategies successfully are the ones who stay sane. BARD suggests that employing such strategies should not be a shameful activity, to be used only when the 'important' tasks have been achieved, but an essential and permanent feature of all consultations. Self-preservation is a professional responsibility for all family doctors.

Who chooses consultation aims?

The chapter on aims offered a considerable list of categories for the potential aims of a family practice consultation. Only some of these aims would be immediately recognised as relevant by most patients, and only some are included in traditional models of the consultation. The chapter went on to suggest that all potential aims deserve consideration, but that there is a limit to what can reasonably be addressed in a single consultation. Patient-centredness would apparently require all of the aims of a consultation to be chosen by the patient involved, but this is not what does happen, not what can happen, nor is it what should happen.

All patients have a limited perspective on the potential aims of a consultation. Those who are non-experts will have an incomplete understanding of treatment or management options, and will need information before informed consent can be obtained. They may have trouble reconciling what they want with what is possible. They will also have limited insight into the other stakeholders in their consultation. Even the patient who is a professor of medicine – clearly not a non-expert – will rely on the third-party problem-solving skills of his family doctor to get a proper scientific perspective on his problem.

A family doctor has a professional responsibility to provide her patients with the information that they need to make choices about the aims that their consultation is to pursue. Patients will generally need help with their choices, and the help they are given and the emphasis that is used will be determined by what the family doctor feels will be in their best interests. A family doctor also has a professional responsibility to have appropriate regard for other stakeholders, and for herself. Few patients will have a complete understanding of the juggling that has to go on in a consultation to keep all of the stakeholders on side. The key is that the family doctor should make her patient aware of which aims are being pursued, so that the aims are on the table for negotiation. BARD assists this process by its emphasis on the nature and use of aims.

Who decides when to stop?

A family doctor with a list of patients to see, and other jobs to do during her working day, clearly has an interest in limiting the time and effort that an individual patient consumes. Other consultation stakeholders will want to see an appropriate compromise reached between the needs of individual patients and the needs of the others who are affected. But are such limits in the interests of patients themselves?

Taking a decision about how much can be dealt with during a single consultation accepts the reality that there is a limit to how much change can be achieved at one sitting. Complex and multiple problems are often better dealt with in segments, especially as time will frequently clarify a situation – there may well be objective advantages to reviewing a patient rather than attempting a 'one-stop' quick fix of everything at once.

Limiting an individual consultation is a way of promoting autonomy, reducing the impact of being a patient, and dealing efficiently with complex problems. It is also a way of sharing resources fairly and recognising the needs of other stakeholders. No family doctor should (so long as safety has been secured) feel guilty about asking a patient to return later to continue the business of a consultation.

For most people, assuming a role as a patient is something to be avoided. It is an admission of loss of control, and an acceptance that treatment (with all the attendant costs in terms of time, money and side-effects) may be needed. Seeking any kind of help from an expert, and taking their advice, represents a loss at least of self-sufficiency if not of autonomy. Attending too many consultations, or having an inappropriately large number of things dealt with as medical problems, reinforces the patient role with all of its drawbacks.

A BARD consultation accepts the limits of what is possible, is open about consultation aims, and does not seek to make people into patients for any longer than is absolutely necessary.

The ethics of acting in a consultation

BARD suggests that family doctors should deliberately choose their behaviour when consulting, and that they should use acting techniques to ensure that their chosen behaviour brings about the intended consultation results. Some family doctors will see this as simply an expression of what is already happening. Others will quite understandably be concerned that by deliberately falsifying her behaviour, a family doctor may not be being honest with her patients. Is such a criticism justified?

Criticism of acting and actors is far from new. Tertullian of Carthage (Quintus Septimus Florens Tertullian, AD 155–222), in his *De Spectaculis*, claimed that acting is inherently immoral because pretending to be someone else involves telling lies. Plato (429–347 BC) would have exiled the acting profession entirely from his ideal *Republic*.

Is acting avoidable?

> All the world's a stage,
> And all the men and women merely players:
> They have their exits and their entrances;
> And each man in his life plays many parts . . .
> Shakespeare, *As You Like It,* II.vii.174

Shakespeare and Goffman[3] are apparently in agreement that, whether they are aware of it or not, all people are putting on an act all of the time. It is no more than an expression of reality to assert that people adjust their behaviour to the circumstances in which they find themselves. It would be neither appropriate nor professional for a family doctor to behave in the same way with her patients as she does, say, with her own children. In her working life, behaviour appropriate for a consultation with a fit woman attending for contraception would not do for an elderly patient who is terminally ill. The reason the behaviour is different is because each encounter has different aims, and those different aims naturally require different elements of behaviour if they are to be achieved.

All forms of behaviour and courtesies have at some point been learned. (There are a limited number of exceptions to this; *see* Chapter 3 on behaviour.) For example, the study of etiquette has in the past formed a substantial part of the education of young people. The novels of Jane Austen and the Brontë sisters from the eighteenth and early nineteenth centuries make much of 'manners' being a fundamental part of polite discourse, and their association with gentility and refinement. The importance of learning how to behave oneself in company is something that our ancestors would be better able to understand than perhaps we can today.

The behaviour on display is the only way by which a person can be judged. The assertion that everyone is acting all the time is, of course, unprovable. How people behave – an observable and measurable phenomenon – may or may not have a close link with what people are thinking or what their intentions are. This link between motivation and action is essentially un-knowable from the outside, as only the person who is having the thoughts can really judge the purpose of the behaviour. People in the outside world can (and will) make assessments of your character based on what you have done, but they can never be sure.

When someone displays inappropriate behaviour, a number of things may have gone wrong. The intention that prompted the behaviour may be inappropriate, and this may well be the interpretation of the behaviour assumed by observers. However, there are other possible reasons. The appropriate behaviour may never have been learned. The behaviour may have been learned, but is displayed incompetently, although it is to be hoped that this will not apply to the BARD family doctor. Alternatively, the circumstances may have been misjudged or interpreted differently so that different behaviour is used.

As Goffman has shown, it is quite possible to explain human social behaviour as a series of 'fronts' or acts that are put on to serve the aims of the moment. It is not necessary to accept this thesis in its entirety to see that looking at behaviour in this way offers insights and perspectives which would not otherwise be available. In the context of a family doctor consultation, if the behaviour is regarded as an act prompted by motivations, then the quality of the act, the quality of the motivation, and the concordance between the two become legitimate areas of study. In addition, it is clear that all of the people – patients and others – who are interacting with the family doctor are also putting on acts in pursuit of their own aims. BARD is saying 'Let's look at consulting as if it were an acting process, and see if that helps us to do things better.' The question therefore is not 'Should a family doctor act during a consultation?' but 'How can the acting be used to get the best result?'.

Is acting dishonest?

When a family doctor deliberately uses behaviour in a consultation to bring about an ulterior objective, does this mean that she is trying to manipulate her patient? Is the consultation simply a game, and the patient a toy?

Acting is only effective if it reflects reality. If the behaviour that an actor used when portraying a role was not consistent with what the audience expect of people in the real world, then that portrayal would not work. In any case, if everyone is constantly acting out a role, reality already consists of acting behaviour. This realisation certainly pre-dates Stanislavsky's 'method' school:

> The only way to arrive at great excellency in characters is to be very conversant with human nature . . . by this way you will more accurately discover the workings of spirit.
>
> David Garrick (1717–1779)

Even when displaying strong emotion, the portrayal that an actor gives is not dishonest. Stanislavsky's ideas about the concept of *emotion memory*[4] require an actor to search his or her own past for examples of behaviour to be used when portraying an emotion dramatically. This means that even though specific behaviour is being used to produce a specific result, that behaviour nevertheless derives from the actor's own life experience. No two actors will portray an emotion in quite the same way – the emotion is real for that actor.

As all actors know, the effect intended by the actor and the effect received by the audience may be quite different. Indeed, one index of success for an actor is that he can deliver what he intends to deliver – the audience shares the joy, sadness, anger, sympathy or whatever. Achieving this result may involve elements of behaviour that do not come naturally. The use of breathing control to support the voice means that everyone in the audience can hear what is happening. Actors tend to speak in complete sentences rather than the little bits and pieces of dialogue interspersed with gaps and 'er' which characterise normal talking. This is not being deceitful – it is simply making the best of the communication opportunities.

No one uses the whole of their behavioural repertoire in every interaction. Some parts of the role that they are portraying are emphasised and other parts are held back. Different patients interacting with a family doctor may well experience different aspects of the family doctor's role. Yet they are experiencing different facets of the same role, not attempts by the family doctor to be someone she is not. To equate such experiences with dishonesty on the part of the family doctor is untenable.

It cannot be assumed that behaviour is more honest if it is intuitive or feels right. Some elements of behaviour inevitably get internalised as a kind of memory shorthand, rather than having to be consciously summoned every time to suit a particular situation. All that this means is that a memory trick has been employed, not that behaviour so confined to the subconscious is any less 'learned' than other behaviour. Habitual behaviour offers a consistent impression to the outside world, so it might be assumed that this truly reflects a person's inner thoughts, or it might just be that this is the behaviour which has brought about the required result in previous similar situations.

Is acting trivial?

The work of a family doctor is never trivial. It is often delightful and sometimes downright hilarious, but it is never trivial. Family doctors are dealing on a daily basis with the essentials of existence – birth and death, and the tricky bit in between which can be characterised by pain or by pleasure. A family doctor is called in at the critical times of life, the times when there is suffering and fear, and when the future may not be as expected. Family doctors are often the harbingers of bad news, and sometimes cause distress. They make fatal diagnoses. They suggest treatments, with all of the attendant inconvenience which that brings. They are becoming increasingly involved with screening procedures, which because of the abundant false-positives are more likely to create anxiety than to reduce disease.

It does not do for a family doctor to be excessively grave and serious. For one thing, being serious all the time is very wearing. For another, most of the work that family doctors involve themselves in does not have a sad outcome – most illnesses get better. It is often appropriate to appear hopeful and optimistic about an outcome, especially as the placebo effect may well be enhanced as a result. In some circumstances, such as work with the depressed, it is absolutely crucial to try and find something to be optimistic about. Improving the social dimension of the relationship with a patient requires the family doctor to appear happy to see him, an emotion that is hard to convey with a frown.

And are we to contrast the seriousness of medical practice with the triviality of acting? Just how trivial a pursuit is acting? At one level, a theatrical performance is an entertainment, a diversion which people choose to attend and share in. You do not go to the theatre to make yourself miserable. Yet merriment and laughter are only some of the reasons why an audience attends. All kinds of emotions can be evoked. New thoughts and ideas are shared. The ability of theatre to explore emotions and relationships – the very fundamentals of the human condition – means that actors are involving themselves in some very serious areas. In what sense could that be described as 'trivial'?

Is acting condescending?

One reason why patients consult with a family doctor is because she is an expert in family medicine – she knows more than her patient and she knows how to use that knowledge. In this respect a consultation is like any other interaction between an expert and a non-expert who wants to use the expert's expertise. It is no more condescending for a family doctor to offer advice to a patient than it is for a plumber to fix your heating or for an electrician to tell you that you have done your wiring all wrong. Experts are expected to know more than you do yourself.

As was argued in Chapter 3 on behaviour, there are times in a family practice consultation when the family doctor may be required to assume the behaviour of higher status. It is a method of emphasising the importance of what is being said. Not to accept this obligation means that the outcome of the consultation may be less good. In the limited context of the job being done, displaying high status is justified. This is not a condescending action, but simply reflects an understanding of the dynamics of a consultation interaction.

The process of reaching a diagnosis, particularly a psychological diagnosis, may be seen as condescending because it requires an ability to express an opinion on what is normal and what is abnormal. The knowledge and process that lead to the making of a diagnosis are unlikely to be understood fully by the patient about whom the opinion is being expressed. Therefore only trained medical practitioners are allowed to say whether people are ill or not. Making a diagnosis is a way of telling the patient that his family doctor knows more about him than he does himself. This process is of course reinforced by the requirement for a medical signature on pieces of paper used for obtaining medicines and financial benefits either from the state or from insurance companies. In some cases, decisions about the presence or absence of illness are particularly politically and socially loaded – for instance, when using the mental health legislation to compulsorily detain a patient. Yet the dilemma is as follows. Even if making a diagnosis can be construed as a condescending act, what precisely is the alternative?

Applying ethical principles

It is suggested that a morally and culturally neutral approach to medical ethics can be achieved by adhering to four principles, and at the same time having due regard to the scope of those principles.[5]

These ethical principles can only be honoured when there is an adequate flow of information from family doctor to patient and from patient to family doctor.

The family doctor needs to know what the patient wants, and vice versa. If the use of acting techniques improves this communication, then such consultations are more likely to be ethically sound.

Respect for autonomy

Patients have a right to have a say in what happens to them – autonomy means 'self-rule'. Patient autonomy can be promoted by making sure that people have all of the relevant information available, so that their consent (or otherwise) can be truly informed. Much medical information is highly technical, so it is also incumbent on the family doctor to acquire the necessary communication skills to present the information in a form that makes sense to the patient. A family doctor who is aware of her role and needs within a consultation is also prompted to be aware of her patient's role and needs, and is thus aware of the information required to ensure that informed consent is obtained.

Patient confidentiality is a promise by the family doctor to keep secrets about patients. Sensitive medical details, which may be essential in order to secure best care, may not be disclosed by patients if the family doctor cannot be trusted to keep her promises. Obtaining all of the facts, and hence suggesting the right management options, requires patients to trust that confidentiality will be respected, so confidentiality is essential to patient autonomy. A family doctor must understand her professional obligations, and behave in a way – by acting if necessary – that secures patient trust.

Autonomy is infringed if patients are deceived by family doctors. BARD is not a dishonest way of practising medicine, and by optimising communication the BARD family doctor is actually less likely to inadvertently deceive a patient. Keeping promises and not deceiving patients works on all levels. For instance, it also implies a requirement to be on time, and the BARD family doctor who understands the role of other stakeholders is more likely to be able to keep to time.

Beneficence

Family doctors should do things that benefit their patients. They should actively promote their patients' interests. The medical consultation is the cornerstone of patient care. If the transfer of information – in both directions – is not of sufficient quality, decisions based on that information will be less than perfect. Strategies that enhance communication during a consultation make a good result more likely.

A BARD consultation will consider all aspects of the patient's life, not just the biomedical aspects. Illness deriving from all sources is likely to be unearthed. A full repertoire of management strategies, including doing nothing, is on offer. And the BARD family doctor will not shirk from her obligation to just be a shoulder to cry on, if that is what the situation requires.

The BARD family doctor will also be very aware of her professional obligation to be medically up to date, to ensure that her patients can be advised of the best management strategies. Also, being conscious of her limitations and the boundaries of her responsibilities, the BARD family doctor is more likely to refer the patient on to medical and other colleagues at the right time. A family doctor who is more aware of the role that she is trying to fulfil will be able to understand when another worker can do the job better.

Non-maleficence

There are many ways in which family doctors can damage their patients. Powerful medications, most of which are poisonous in the wrong doses, are prescribed many times each working day. Patients are assaulted with needles and prodded in deep and secret places. Sensitive and embarrassing information is disclosed. Family doctors are allowed to ask questions and to do things to patients which those patients would not permit from anybody else. It is a privilege to be allowed such access, but also a fearsome responsibility.

The principle of non-maleficence must be balanced against the principle of beneficence. It is not sufficient to do nothing just in case something goes wrong. Doing nothing may often be in the patient's best interests, so long as his family doctor has been able to explain convincingly just why she proposes to do nothing. On the other hand, a family doctor who does nothing just to save herself from the courts or the medical regulatory authority is not behaving ethically.

Working out a patient management strategy that will deliver overall benefit must take into account more than the strictly biomedical. Some hypertensive patients will decide to take their chances untreated rather than suffer the erectile dysfunction that the tablets cause – others will not. The BARD family doctor's potential consultation aims are wide-ranging, and allow that for each consultation and decision there are legitimate competing interests. The correct management of a problem is not something that only the family doctor can or ought to try to define. This can be viewed as another way of respecting patient autonomy – at the end of the day, the patient has the final say.

Justice

Family doctors should treat their patients fairly. This includes making sure that they get a fair share of treatments, that their rights are respected, and that they are treated according to morally acceptable laws. Treating people fairly is not the same as treating them identically. As Aristotle pointed out some time ago, people can be treated unjustly even if they are treated equally. A family doctor exercises justice by treating her patients according to need, and according to who will benefit.

Yet who is to assess need? Who is to balance the priorities of the individual against society or the health services? The BARD family doctor is adept at such juggling, at 'muddling through elegantly'.[6] She recognises the legitimacy of the different stakeholders – patients, the healthcare system, the state – and tries to make the best of things while at the same time actively promoting her patient's interests. To bend Virchow a little, medicine is just like politics, but on a smaller scale.[8.1]

The BARD family doctor, by exercising her superior communication techniques, is better placed to determine patient needs and also better able to appreciate her patient's perception of need.

[8.1] Rudolph Virchow actually said 'Medicine is a social science, and politics nothing but medicine on a grand scale.'

Scope

The final requirement is to decide who these four principles should apply to. Superficially this is quite an easy problem for a family doctor – clearly the principles should apply to her patients. But, for instance, does autonomy apply to all patients? What about children? What about the mentally impaired? The autonomy to choose what to eat or what to wear is of a different order to that concerning decisions about serious medical procedures, so is autonomy allowed for some decisions but not for others? Is the balance of beneficence and non-maleficence the same for a child as for a pensioner, or for a disabled patient as for a non-disabled one?

A family doctor who has thought through her role and its implications will have a much better idea of how to reconcile such issues. As well as being aware of her obligations, she will also be aware of the limits of those obligations, and so free of the anxiety of underachievement. The family doctor who is disabled by anxiety disadvantages all of her patients. When decisions about patient care are better taken by politicians, managers, economists, ethicists or lawyers, then for the BARD family doctor medical arrogance does not intrude – no one has a monopoly of the truth.

Summary

Because it is different, and because it draws on inspiration from outside the medical profession, BARD might be regarded as unethical. However, the application of BARD is entirely consistent with patient-centred consulting, and possibly more so than traditional consulting models allow. It is not deceitful, trivial or condescending. The application of an established set of medical ethical principles confirms that the BARD practitioner can consult with confidence and enthusiasm in the certain knowledge that she is upholding the ethical as well as the medical best interests of her patients.

References

1. Freeman G, Carr J and Hill A (2004) The journey towards patient-centredness. *Br J Gen Pract.* **54**: 651–2.
2. Smith R (2003) Thoughts for new medical students at a new medical school. *BMJ.* **327**: 1430–3.
3. Goffman E (1990) *The Presentation of Self in Everyday Life.* Penguin, Harmondsworth.
4. Morrison H (1998) *Acting Skills* (2e). A & C Black, London.
5. Gillon R (1994) Medical ethics: four principles plus attention to scope. *BMJ.* **309**: 184–8.
6. Hunter DJ (1993) *Rationing Dilemmas in Health Care.* National Association of Health Authorities and Trusts, Birmingham.

Index